Cardiovascular Physiology

A Clinical Approach

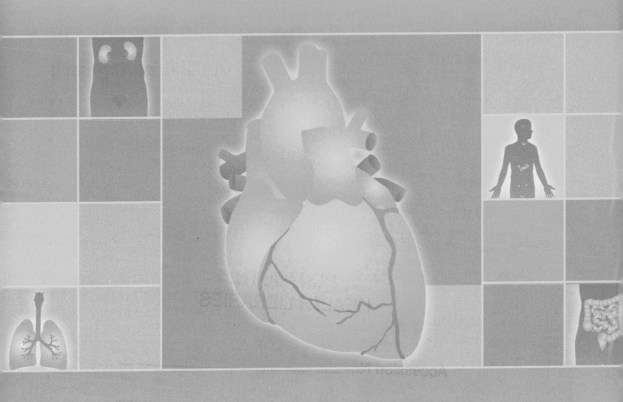

Cardiovascular Physiology
A Clinical Approach

Carol-Ann Courneya, PhD
Associate Professor
Department of Cellular and Physiological Sciences
Faculty Medicine
The University of British Columbia
Vancouver, BC, Canada

Michael J. Parker, MD
Assistant Professor of Medicine
Division of Pulmonary and Critical Care Medicine
Beth Israel Deaconess Medical Center
Senior Interactive Media Architect
Center for Educational Technology
Harvard Medical School
Boston, MA

Series Editor
Richard M. Schwartzstein, MD
Director
Harvard Medical School Academy
Ellen and Melvin Gordon Professor of Medicine and Medical Education
Harvard Medical School
Vice President for Education
Beth Israel Deaconess Medical Center
Boston, MA

Wolters Kluwer | Lippincott Williams & Wilkins
Health
Philadelphia · Baltimore · New York · London
Buenos Aires · Hong Kong · Sydney · Tokyo

Acquisitions Editor: Crystal Taylor
Product Manager: Kelley Squazzo
Marketing Manager: Brian Moody
Vendor Manager: Bridgett Dougherty
Manufacturing Manager: Margie Orzech-Zeranko
Design Coordinator: Doug Smock
Compositor: Aptara, Inc.

First Edition

Copyright © 2011 Lippincott Williams & Wilkins, a Wolters Kluwer business.

351 West Camden Street   Two Commerce Square
Baltimore, MD 21201   2001 Market Street
                                Philadelphia, PA 19103

Printed in China

9   8   7   6   5   4   3   2   1

Library of Congress Cataloging-in-Publication Data

Courneya, Carol Ann Margaret, 1957-
  Cardiovascular physiology : a clinical approach / Carol-Ann Courneya,
Michael J. Parker. – 1st ed.
     p. ; cm. – (Integrated physiology series)
  Includes bibliographical references and index.
  ISBN 978-0-7817-7485-7 (alk. paper)
  1. Cardiovascular system–Physiology.   I. Parker, Michael J.   II.
Title.   III. Series: Integrated physiology series.
  [DNLM: 1. Cardiovascular Physiological Phenomena.   WG 102 C861 2011]
  QP101.C84 2011
  612.1–dc22

                                        2010002040

DISCLAIMER

*To my father Joseph, and to the memory of my mother Florence (1922–2008),
for it was you who provided the foundation for my learning. I also dedicate this
book to my husband David Dunne whose love supports me and
whose talent as an educator inspires me.*

—CAC

*To my wonderful wife, Yuanzhen, and my parents, Leonard and Gloria:
for being there with endless support, enthusiasm, and love.*

—MJP

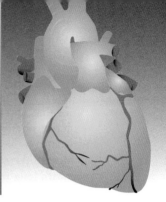

Preface

Introduction

The goal of *Cardiovascular Physiology: A Clinical Approach* is to provide a clear, clinically oriented exposition of the essentials of cardiovascular physiology for medical students, residents, nurses, and allied health professionals. We present the physiology in the context of a system to emphasize that the functions we associate with the circulation depend on more than the heart. This approach is essential for a complete understanding of the clinical problems that affect the heart and blood vessels and that lead to symptoms of ischemic chest pain, hypotension, and heart failure.

This book is the second in *The Integrated Physiology Series*, a sequence of monographs on physiology. The first book, *Respiratory Physiology: A Clinical Approach*, describes the essential principles underlying breathing. Additional books in development at this time will address renal and gastrointestinal function. Each book will be designed to meet the needs of the learners outlined below and will use the same style and pedagogical tools. In addition, we have attempted to design common frameworks upon which the student can hang the large amounts of information confronting us in medicine today and with which a foundation can be built to support the incorporation of new knowledge in the future. In this book, for example, we describe the cardiovascular system in the context of the controller (the regulation of heart rate, contractility, and vascular tone), the pump function (the determinants of stroke volume and cardiac output), and the exchanger (the distribution of blood to the tissue and the exchange of oxygen, carbon dioxide, nutrients, and the products of metabolism). This same framework—controller, pump, and exchanger—is applicable to the respiratory system and used in the first book of the series. Thus, learning concepts important for one organ system will facilitate understanding when you study the other organ system. The series addresses "integrated" physiology by its focus on systems rather than on organs and by making explicit links between systems.

Our goals are to present physiology in a clinically meaningful way, to emphasize that physiology is best understood within the context of an organ *system*, to demonstrate principles that are common to different systems, and to utilize an interactive style that engages and challenges the reader.

Level

The level of the book is intended to fit a range of needs from students who have had no previous exposure to physiology to residents who are now in the thick of patient care but feel the need to review relevant physiology in a clinical context. We have drawn upon many years of experience teaching students, residents, and fellows in making decisions with respect to the topics emphasized and the clinical examples used to illustrate key concepts. The book is not intended as a comprehensive review of cardiovascular physiology nor is it designed for the advanced, research-oriented physiologist. Rather, we have focused on issues that are most relevant for the care of patients while, at the same time, we provide sufficient physiological detail to provide you with the foundation to examine and analyze new data on these topics in the future.

Most of the concepts presented in the book are well established and we do not burden you with long reference lists for this information. When we present newer and, in some cases, more controversial issues, however, we do provide relevant primary source citations.

Content

The book begins with two chapters that serve to provide context for the study of cardiovascular physiology. In Chapter 1, we layout the framework (controller, pump, and exchanger) of the cardiovascular system upon which we will hang concepts and information in the succeeding chapters. In the process of building this framework, we also give you an opportunity to experience some of the interactive elements of the text that will be revisited in subsequent chapters. Chapter 2 focuses on functional anatomy, linking the essential elements of the structure of the cardiovascular system to their physiological role.

In the next two chapters (3 and 4), we address the heart as a pump, first examining the cellular physiology underlying contraction and then taking a macroscopic view of the function of the heart as an organ comprising muscle and valves. Chapters 5 and 6 center on the controller, the combination of central and local factors that affect the rate and rhythm of the heart.

Chapters 7 and 8 bring us back to the heart as a pump and focus on the principles essential to the understanding of cardiac output, and the blood vessels that distribute the output to the appropriate tissues under different metabolic conditions. In addition, Chapter 8 addresses the exchanger, the capillaries across which gases, nutrients, and wastes move from the vascular space to the tissues and back again; we also focus on factors that determine the movement of fluid across capillaries and the formation of edema. In Chapter 9, we present an integration chapter that brings together concepts essential for the understanding of blood pressure control. Finally, in Chapter 10, we integrate all of the elements of the cardiovascular system by examining the physiology of pregnancy.

For those interested in a detailed look at the cardiovascular system during exercise, we refer you to Chapter 9 of the first book in the series, *Respiratory Physiology: A Clinical Approach*. In that chapter, we examine exercise by taking an integrated approach to the adaptive responses of both the respiratory and cardiovascular systems.

Throughout this book, we draw heavily upon clinical examples to emphasize concepts and to highlight how an understanding of normal physiological principles will help you understand pathological states. For the beginning student, you will see the relevance of the material presented. For the advanced student or resident, these examples will help you understand the signs and symptoms of your patients and the rationale for therapeutic interventions.

Pedagogy

The following teaching elements are common to all of the books in the *Integrated Physiology Series*

- **Chapter Outline.** The outline at the beginning of each chapter gives a preview of the chapter and is a useful study aid.
- **Learning Objectives.** Each chapter starts with a short list of learning objectives. These objectives are intended to help you focus on the most critical concepts and physiological principles that will be presented in the chapter.

- **Text.** The text is written in a conversational style that is intended to recreate the sense of participating in an interactive lecture. Questions are posed periodically to offer you opportunities to reflect on information presented and to try your hand at synthesizing and applying your knowledge to novel situations.
- **Topic Headings.** Topic headings are used to delineate key concepts. Sections are arranged to present the material in easily digestible quantities as you move from simple to more complex physiology.
- **Boldfacing.** Key terms are boldfaced at their first appearance in a chapter. Definitions for all boldfaced terms are found in the glossary.
- **Thought Questions.** Interposed within the text are *thought questions* that are designed to challenge you to use the material just presented in the text in a novel fashion. Many of these are posed in a clinical context to demonstrate the clinical relevance of the material as well.
- **Editor's Integration.** Periodically in the text you will notice a box that makes a link between a concept in one organ system with the same or very similar concept in another organ system. This information will help reinforce knowledge in both areas and illustrate further the ways in which physiology can be integrated.
- **Illustrations and Animated Figures.** The figures have been developed to demonstrate the relationship between physiological variables, to illustrate key concepts, and to integrate a number of principles enumerated in the text. Many of the figures in this book are linked to interactive learning tools (called "Animated Figures" in the text) that will provide you with an opportunity to view a physiological principle in motion or to manipulate variables and see the physiological consequences of the changes. These animations and computer simulations permit the reader to work with the concepts and to apply them in a range of circumstances. Our goal is that, with self-paced use of these interactive animations, you will gain a deeper, more intuitive, understanding of the physiological principles discussed in each chapter.
- **Tables and Boxed Lists.** Tables and boxed lists provide summaries of information outlined in the text.
- **"Putting It together" section.** At the end of each chapter is a clinical case presentation that poses questions about physical findings, laboratory values, or diagnostic and therapeutic issues that can be answered with the physiological information presented in the chapter. These cases are designed to integrate material, to demonstrate the clinical relevance of the physiology, and to provide you with an opportunity to test yourself by applying what you have just learned in a new situation.
- **Review Questions and Answers.** You can use the review questions at the end of each chapter to test whether you have mastered the material. For medical students, the USMLE-type questions should help you prepare for the Step 1 examination. Answers to the questions are presented at the end of the book and include explanations that delineate why the choices are correct or incorrect.
- **Index.** A complete index allows you to easily find material in the text.

In the final analysis, most people study physiology because it offers great insights into the workings of the human body. We have organized and presented the material in this book in a way that we hope will allow you to achieve your individual goals while having some fun with a subject that continues to challenge and intrigue us.

Richard M. Schwartzstein, MD
Ellen and Melvin Gordon Professor of Medicine and Medical Education
Harvard Medical School
Editor, *The Integrated Physiology Series*

Acknowledgments

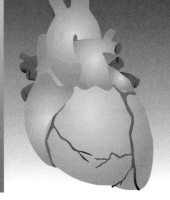

The creation of this book is an endeavor to which many have contributed. This is our opportunity as authors to express our appreciation to the people who have supported us behind the scenes, and to those who have collaborated with us and inspired us.

At Lippincott Williams & Wilkins, we are grateful to Nancy Hoffmann, who was our initial managing editor, and to Kelley Squazzo and Crystal Taylor for helping bring this book to fruition. In her role as agent, Liz Allison has been absolutely vital to the success of this project, helping us always move things forward.

We thank our editor Dr. Richard Schwartzstein for his diligence, patience, and unflagging sense of humor, as well as his pedagogical wisdom; he truly cares about teaching, and his guidance has helped immensely in shaping this book.

I (CAC) thank Drs. Len Lilly, William Ovalle, and Wayne Vogl who wrote such amazing books and set the bar so high; Dr. Ovalle for sharing with me his unbridled joy for teaching; Dr. Jason Waechter who is a model of teaching clinically relevant cardiac science and who provided me with many clinical examples for "thought questions" in this book; Dr. Ed Moore whose explanations of EC coupling informed Chapter 3; Dr. Eric Accili who guided me to a deeper understanding of cardiac potassium channels; Dr. Steve Yau who found time during a busy residency program to create review questions for this text, Dr. Robert Woollard for his friendship and sage advice, and the CV block captains at UBC (Drs. Waechter, Cairns, Finkler, Patterson, and Bailey) who make teaching cardiac science so much fun. I thank my coauthor Dr. Michael Parker for joining me on this academic journey and sharing his astounding creativity in animation. I thank my past students (you will know who you are) because it was you I imagined I was talking to as I wrote about these various topics. I thank my Nepalese colleagues whose unswerving commitment to medical education is humbling. I would like to warmly acknowledge the Wilson Centre in Toronto, Canada, for providing me with a sabbatical home for writing this book.

I (MJP) am grateful to those who have inspired and supported me in my chosen path of teaching, writing, and creating interactive tools to help students visualize and understand difficult concepts in medicine. John Halamka, MD, has been a steadfast supporter of the development of animations and simulations in the Harvard curriculum and has been encouraging in the efforts to build on that foundation for this book. John shares the vision for educational innovation, and that is something I truly appreciate. For me, Rich Schwartzstein's influence extends beyond his role as editor; he has been a valuable collaborator through much of my career in medicine and teaching. I thank Carol Ann, my coauthor, for the enthusiasm and endless positive energy she has brought to this project; her sense of humor in tolerating the perfectionistic streak in me has been invaluable. I would also like to warmly express gratitude to Thomas Rocco, MD, who has helped and inspired me in many ways; his vast knowledge of the cardiovascular system is only part of that. His encouragement, support, and friendship have meant a great deal to me.

Finally, we would like to thank those closest to us. I (CAC) would like to thank my family (Gerry & Jill, Bill & Nancy, Chris, Michelle & Jack, Angie & Danny, and Geoff & Jen), my wonderful loving friends in Vancouver and Toronto, and my wise father "Joe Primeau" for all your combined love and support. And a loving thank you to David for your endless creativity and thoughtfulness. I (MJP) would like to thank my parents, whose enthusiasm, curiosity, and love of learning have provided the best inspiration a person could possibly have. Thank you to my wife Yuanzhen: your support, humor, patience, and wisdom bring out the best in me.

Contents

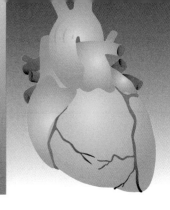

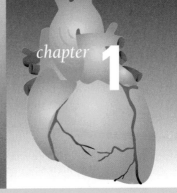

chapter 1

Getting Started:
The Approach to Cardiovascular Physiology

CHAPTER OUTLINE

LEARNING OBJECTIVES

By the end of the chapter you will be able to:
- **Delineate the principles that support the concept that cardiovascular physiology must be studied within the context of the cardiovascular system.**
- **Outline the elements of the cardiac system.**
- **Delineate the learning tools that will be used throughout this book.**
- **Describe the best methods for use of the learning tools contained within this book.**

Introduction

Although there will always be debate among specialists as to the organs that are the most essential to life, it would be hard not to see the heart at or near the top of the list. No heart, no blood being pumped and, therefore, no oxygen and nutrient delivery to the other organs. In addition to its biological importance, philosophers have, at times in the past, described the heart as the seat of the soul.

The study of the physiology of the cardiovascular system is relevant for all medical specialties from internal medicine to surgery to psychiatry. An understanding of acute and chronic cardiovascular disease is critical for all physicians providing clinical care. The multiple factors that can interfere with the normal circulation cut across specialties. The unique blend of automatic and behavioral control of the heart rate, for example, creates linkages between human behavior and cardiovascular physiology. If you plan on entering the field of psychiatry some day, you may be confronted with a patient with panic attacks, palpitations, and a series of symptoms that can best be understood within the context of cardiovascular physiology.

When you heard you were about to study cardiovascular physiology, chances are that your first thought was "I will be studying the heart." Although the heart is clearly an essential element of the processes that account for the circulation, it alone does not provide the whole story. Rather, one must step back and look at the vascular system, which is responsible for distributing the blood to and collecting it from the various organs in the body, and the microscopic vessels that determine the exchange of oxygen, carbon dioxide, and nutrients that sustain life. Consider that without skeletal muscles in the legs and valves in the leg veins, it would be difficult to promote the return of blood from the body (against gravity) back to the heart. The medulla, the region of the brainstem that monitors blood pressure and sends appropriately timed neurological impulses via the autonomic nervous system to the heart and blood vessels, is essential for simple activities, such as going from a lying to sitting position, as well as for complex processes, such as exercise. As you proceed from one chapter to another, we will periodically orient you to where we are in the cardiovascular system and show you how the different components interact.

Physiology is, at its core, a conceptual science. The study of physiology is critical to understanding the way in which the body functions and the many mechanisms available to restore homeostasis when disease attacks. Our goal throughout this book is to emphasize conceptual understanding of the material. We want you to develop an appreciation for physiological principles at a depth sufficient to allow you to apply the concepts to new situations, thereby enabling you to make sense of a unique patient, the ultimate challenge in medicine. Our emphasis is on clinical physiology. Given the great range of information that physicians in training must learn, we emphasize those principles that are most essential for you to care for patients and that provide a strong foundation upon which to build as you go on to more advanced levels of study. Although we use clinical examples throughout the text to demonstrate the relevance of the material and the ways in which the concepts are applied to patients, **this is a physiology,** *not* **pathophysiology, book.** Thus, we will not be describing in detail specific disease states, diagnostic methods, or treatment options, except as they may enhance your understanding of the physiology. Given the emphasis on this clinical approach, we will not spend considerable time on some physiological points found in classic texts that are neither clinically relevant nor necessary to have a solid foundation in the field. We acknowledge that this is not a text aimed primarily at the basic science physiologist. Rather, we are striving to provide the clinical physiologist with the essential information needed for patient care today, and the understanding to add to that fund of knowledge in the future.

Much of what we know about physiology derives from careful observations of people and of animal models. From these observations, hypotheses have been constructed to help explain the findings. In some cases, hypotheses have been tested extensively and modified accordingly. In other situations, we are still working largely at the level of conjecture. For those of you who have a need for definitive answers in all circumstances, you may be frustrated at times in your study of physiology. The "proof" is not always available to us. Perhaps you may be intrigued by one of these areas of uncertainty and pursue further investigations yourself to provide us all with greater insights into the workings of the human body.

This book is designed primarily for medical students who are embarking upon the study of cardiovascular physiology for the first time, but it will also serve as an excellent review for advanced medical students, interns, and residents, especially for those whose initial instruction in cardiovascular physiology took a more traditional basic science approach to the subject. The field of physiology changes rapidly and this book will provide you with up-to-date concepts as they relate to clinical practice. Nurses and cardiac therapists who care for patients with cardiac problems may also find this text very useful. This book is not intended as a definitive or all-encompassing resource on cardiac physiology. Those pursuing advanced training in cardiology and critical care medicine or anesthesiology may rely upon this as a primer as they expand their knowledge into the subtleties of the field.

Cardiovascular Physiology

A SYSTEMS APPROACH

In teaching physiology to medical students for the past decade, we have often heard a plaintiff plea for assistance in making the different things they were learning "fit together." For knowledge to be both meaningful and useful, it is important to have a superstructure upon which to hang individual concepts. Similarly, in teaching interns and residents for the past 20 years, we have seen many mistakes made in the care of patients with cardiac disease because of the exclusive focus on the heart as the doctor tried to analyze the problem at hand. The answer to both of these problems is a systems approach to cardiovascular physiology.

The cardiovascular system comprises all of the elements needed to move freshly oxygenated blood from the heart to various organs, through a vast network of capillaries, for exchange of oxygen and carbon dioxide, and finally back to the heart and to the lungs to pick up fresh oxygen and off-load carbon dioxide. The core components of this system are the cardiac controller, the pump, and the exchanger. The cardiac controller consists of the elements of the central nervous system that tell the heart how fast and how hard to beat (e.g., medulla, hypothalamus, and higher cortical centers) and assists in regulation of the peripheral vasculature, a function critical to maintaining blood pressure and ensuring that blood is directed to the most metabolically active tissues; the intrinsic electrical system of the heart is also a component of the controller. The system to which we refer as "the pump" consists of four chambers of cardiac muscle (separated by one-way valves), whose coordinated contraction propels the blood to the lungs and to the rest of the body, and the blood vessels, which serve as the conduit for the flow of blood to and from the capillaries. The third component of the system, the exchanger, comprises the capillaries across which oxygen, carbon dioxide, nutrients, and metabolic products are exchanged in every tissue in the body. In the lungs, fresh oxygen is taken up into the pulmonary capillaries and exchanged for the carbon dioxide that was generated by the tissues. The remaining capillaries in the cardiovascular system (distributed within all the other organs of the body) operate in reverse—oxygen is transported to the tissues and carbon dioxide is moved to the alveoli (*Figure* 1-1).

EDITOR'S INTEGRATION
There are many concepts in cardiovascular physiology that are common to respiratory physiology as well. For example, you will be learning about the factors that govern flow through tubes and diffusion of oxygen and carbon dioxide across capillaries. To assist you in understanding the concepts that will help you with both organ systems, we have setup a common framework for organizing the material—controller, pump, and exchanger. The respiratory system has a controller that regulates how rapidly and deeply you breathe, a pump that moves gas into and out of your lungs, and a gas exchanger across which oxygen and carbon dioxide diffuse.

As we proceed on our journey, we will begin with an overview of the anatomy of the cardiac system, emphasizing the form and function of the anatomic structures (Chapter 2). From there, we begin our study of the pump by examining the important link between electrical stimulation or excitation of cardiac muscle cells and the transformation of that excitation into cardiac contraction—this is called "excitation–contraction coupling" (Chapter 3). The process that ultimately leads to pumping blood from the heart to the

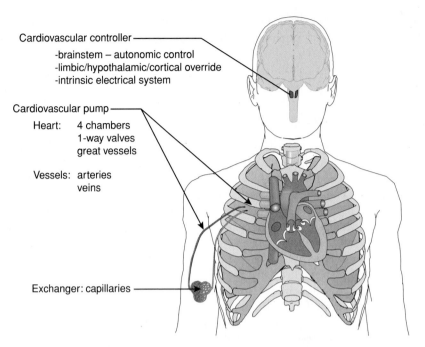

Cardiovascular controller
    -brainstem – autonomic control
    -limbic/hypothalamic/cortical override
    -intrinsic electrical system

Cardiovascular pump
   Heart: 4 chambers
               1-way valves
               great vessels

   Vessels: arteries
                 veins

Exchanger: capillaries

FIGURE 1-1 The components of the cardiovascular system.

lungs and to the body requires exquisite orchestration of electrical and physical events. Chapter 4 describes this sequence of events, known as the "cardiac cycle," through one complete phase of cardiac pumping (called systole) and relaxation (called diastole). The cardiac cycle integrates several concepts: the determinants of blood flow through the heart, the relationship between pressure in the heart chambers and the operation of the cardiac valves, the initiation and progression of the electrical stimulus, and the correlation between mechanical events in the heart and sounds you hear when you listen to the heart with a stethoscope.

In Chapter 5, we begin our examination of the cardiovascular system's controller by describing the intrinsic pacemakers within the heart, the wiring that links all cardiac cells together electrically, and the role of the brain and autonomic nervous system in regulating the pacemaker cells. One of the most clinically useful, noninvasive cardiac tests is the electrocardiograph (or ECG), which reflects the electrical activity of the heart. In Chapter 6, we describe the elements necessary for generating, and beginning to interpret, the basic waveforms (called the P, QRS, and T waves) that constitute the ECG, and link the mechanical actions of the cardiac pump with the underlying electrical stimuli responsible for those actions.

The ultimate measure of heart function is the volume of blood it pumps every minute, called the "cardiac output." In Chapter 7, we return to our discussion of the pump by elaborating the determinants of cardiac output (the factors that alter the rate of cardiac contraction and the amount of blood ejected with each beat), including discussions about the role of the brain and autonomic nervous system in determining how fast and forcefully the heart contracts. A complete understanding of cardiac output requires that you also know how the blood is delivered to and apportioned among the various organs of the body. We tackle this topic in Chapter 8 on blood vessels, in which we describe the various types and roles of blood vessels and link the pump to the exchanger component of the cardiovascular system. We talk about the distinction between transport, distribution, and capacitance vessels, and the special requirements that must be met for the exchange of gases and nutrients.

It would be rare these days to find a person who does not know someone being treated for "high blood pressure." Just what is blood pressure? What defines whether blood pressure is "too high" or "too low?" How is blood pressure controlled? These are questions we will tackle in Chapter 9. In the final chapter (Chapter 10), we bring all the key cardiovascular components together in our discussion of the cardiovascular adaptations associated with pregnancy. In order to accommodate a growing fetus, the cardiovascular system within the female body undergoes many changes. Blood volume is dramatically expanded, hormone levels fluctuate, new blood vessels are formed, and the tone of the existing blood vessels is changed. All of this leads up to the drama of labor and delivery, which requires its own set of cardiovascular adjustments, and then, shortly after birth, everything returns to the way it was before the pregnancy. In our discussion of pregnancy, we hope to provide you with an opportunity to integrate the material from Chapters 2 through 9.

As we develop the concepts in each of these chapters, we will continually bring you back to the superstructure of the cardiovascular system—controller, pump, exchanger—so you will understand how the individual pieces fit together. To assist you in learning the terminology of physiology, we will highlight new terms and provide definitions in a glossary at the end of the text.

A CLINICAL APPROACH

Given the vast quantities of information confronting doctors today, most students and residents want to know why a new piece of knowledge is essential for them to master. Why should I learn this? As a general principle, the answer to this question has two components. First, this knowledge will enable you to take better care of your patients today and in the future. Second, the construction of this foundation or framework will help you incorporate new knowledge about human function and disease as it is discovered in the future.

To help you see the relevance of cardiovascular physiology, we place the study of this subject within a clinical context as much as possible. We draw upon clinical examples to reinforce and clarify concepts. At the end of each chapter, we provide a section called "Putting It Together" in which we present a brief clinical scenario that illustrates many of the principles of the chapter and further reinforces the concepts just developed. Thus, the question of relevance will be addressed in a very explicit manner.

The Keys to the Vault: Helping You Master This Material

Critical thinking—as teachers, we want our students to be able to do it; as students you hope to be able to demonstrate it. To think critically about physiology and your patients, you must be able to understand concepts, not merely so they can be repeated back to the teacher in a rote fashion, but in a way that they can be applied to new situations. To do this, one needs to achieve a level of understanding that is more than skin deep; one needs to have an intuitive feel for the concepts and their implications for the body's function. You must be able to manipulate the principles, so they can shed insight on puzzles and open doors to help you find the way out of the maze. To help you achieve this goal, we have taken an approach that is more conceptual than quantitative. We emphasize the equations and calculations you will need as a clinician, and otherwise utilize numbers when it will enhance understanding rather than distract from it. We have provided a number of learning tools that are intended to help you develop the depth of understanding necessary for you to be able to think critically as a clinical physiologist.

ANIMATED FIGURES

To give you a chance to work with the concepts developed in the text, you will have opportunities to try your hand at a variety of computer-based animations and simulations (directions for accessing these can be found inside the book's cover). These interactive diagrams are designed to allow you to view an animation of a concept, or to manipulate, at your own pace, a number of variables that change over a range of physiologic conditions. You can experiment by changing parameters, predict the consequences of these changes, and then puzzle over which principles accounted for the transition from the first condition to the second. For those students who are visual learners (and for those of you who believe in the aphorism that "one picture is worth a thousand words"), we hope these learning opportunities will enhance the text. In certain cases, we provide simultaneous auditory, textual, and animated material to engage your senses in the learning experience.

In some of the more complex Animated Figures, we suggest that you focus on one aspect of the animation at a time, and then sit back and see if you can integrate everything that is happening at once. In essence, focus on one part of the puzzle and then another until the entire picture reveals itself to you. For example, take a look at Animated Figure 1-1 (Cardiac cycle integration). There is much going on here. When you play the animation, the heart contracts and relaxes, and you see the heart valves opening and closing; all of this is synchronized with an audio recording of the heart sounds. At the same time, you are looking at graphs of how pressure and volume change in the left ventricle, the major pumping chamber of the heart, over the cardiac cycle. The tracing of the electrical activity of the heart gives a hint of what you will see when you study how the cardiac conduction system coordinates the contraction of the heart. What mechanical events are associated with the first and second heart sounds? What is the timing of electrical activity of the heart in relation to pressure changes? You will need to ask yourself questions like these when using the diagrams with the text. In certain cases, the text will pose these questions to you, guiding your use of the figure. Such a diagram may seem a bit overwhelming to you right now, but as you progress through the chapters, the concepts depicted will become clear to you.

THOUGHT QUESTIONS

In the early 20th century, the world-renowned physicist Albert Einstein created "gedanken experiments," or thought experiments, to help him analyze the forces of the universe. These were experimental situations that he worked through intellectually rather than physically to find fallacies in his reasoning. In the spirit of Einstein, we have interspersed thought questions throughout the text to assist you in working through concepts and principles of cardiovascular physiology. We urge you to take the time to ponder the thought questions when they arise, since they are strategically placed to reinforce the concepts developed up to that point in the text and Animated Figures. Thus, an inability to answer the thought question should prompt you to revisit the material that precedes it.

? **THOUGHT QUESTION 1-1: When astronauts are thrust from earth into space and away from the confines of gravity, what key changes might you expect in the way blood flows around the circulatory system? What nervous or hormonal reflexes might be triggered?**

Answers to the thought questions can be found at the end of each chapter.

REVIEW QUESTIONS

At the end of each chapter, we have placed a number of review questions that will enable you to do a self-assessment of your learning. The questions are based on mini-case time course than the fast sodium channel current we saw in non-pacemaker cells) leads to the slow upstroke once the voltage has reached the threshold to initiate an AP. We will revisit the shape of the pacemaker action potential later in the chapter when we examine other potential sources of pacemaker activity in the heart as well as the effects of the autonomic nervous system on heart rate.

Refractory Period

As we discussed in Chapter 5, the ion channels that are responsible for the rapid upstroke of action potential (phase 0) go through a sequence of states from closed to open to inactivated and back to closed. The membrane voltage plays a large role in determining the probability that the channels will be in each state. For example, most fast sodium channels in ventricular cells are in the closed state at the very negative voltages that are seen at or near the resting membrane potential. It is not until the cell begins to depolarize, and the voltage becomes less negative (or more positive), that the fast sodium channels open. Quickly, however, as the cell depolarizes, they become inactivated. The process of repolarization, which reestablishes a negative transmembrane potential, moves the sodium channels from an inactivated to a closed state and, thereby, prepares them to reopen. During the time the fast sodium channels are inactivated, they are not available to reopen and, thus, a new action potential cannot be stimulated. This period is called the **refractory period** because the cell is unable to generate a new action potential when current is received from the depolarization of an adjacent cell; it is refractory or resistant to the electrical stimulus.

The initial portion of the refractory period is called the absolute refractory period because all sodium channels are in the inactivated state. As the membrane repolarizes during phase 3, however, some sodium channels pass through the inactivated state to a closed state and become available to open again. The time interval from the beginning of repolarization, at which point sodium channels begin to resume the closed state, until the cell returns to its resting membrane potential, and essentially all sodium channels are closed, is called the relative refractory period; the arrival of current from an adjacent cell during the relative refractory period causes a weak electrical response that might trigger a second action potential (*Figure* 5-4)

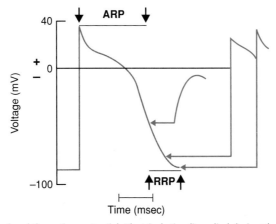

FIGURE 5-4 Refractory period and the action potential. Electrical stimuli applied during the absolute refractory period (ARP) do not result in the production of a new action potential. Stimuli during the relative refractory period (RRP), however, can produce weak or incomplete action potentials. The absolute refractory period protects the heart from tetanic contractions, which would rapidly be life threatening.

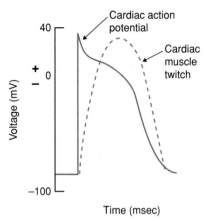

FIGURE 5-5 Action potential and twitch duration. In this figure you can see a ventricular cell action potential with a mechanical muscle twitch (hatched line) superimposed on the same timeline. It is easy to see that their durations are almost identical. Because of the presence of the refractory period, the muscle is protected electrically from accepting an electrical stimulus until it is mechanically relaxed. Consequently, multiple, closely timed electrical stimuli cannot cause the ventricular muscle to go into a tetanic contraction. Adapted from Rhoades RA and Bell DR. *Medical Physiology: Principles for Clinical Medicine.* 3rd ed. Baltimore, MD: Lippincott Williams & Wilkins, 2009; 244. Figure 13-1.

     Use Animated Figure 5-4 (Refractory period) to see how the states of the sodium channels relate to the absolute refractory period (during which no action potential can be generated) and the relative refractory period (during which a stronger than normal stimulus can initiate an action potential, albeit one that is slower conducting and lower in amplitude). Try stimulating the cell during different portions of the action potential and see what the resulting depolarization (when there is one) looks like.

In skeletal muscle, the duration of a nerve action potential is 2 to 3 msec, whereas the twitch duration is hundreds of milliseconds long. If repetitive electrical stimuli are delivered to the muscle prior to completion of mechanical contraction, the effect is a sustained contraction with no repolarization, a condition known as "tetany." You can imagine how disastrous that would be were it to occur in cardiac muscle. There would be a prolonged single contraction and no cardiac output. The human heart, fortunately, has evolved in a way to prevent tetany from occurring. In cardiac muscle, in contrast to skeletal muscle, the duration of the ventricular cell AP is much longer (~200 msec) and, more importantly, the absolute refractory period is approximately equal to the duration of a ventricular muscle cell twitch (*Figure 5-5*).

The presence of the absolute refractory period throughout twitch duration prevents tetanic contraction in the heart. By the time the next possible AP can be generated, the muscle has almost fully relaxed, has filled with blood, and can eject blood to the body. Thus, repetitive electrical stimuli do not produce sustained contraction of the cardiac muscle; a second contraction cannot be triggered until mechanical relaxation has occurred.

The Electrical Conduction System

ATRIAL CONDUCTION PATHWAY

Having initiated electrical signals in the SA node, the system needs to distribute them rapidly to other parts of the heart to generate an effective contraction. First, one must get current rapidly through the atria. The current generated by the APs in the pacemaker cells

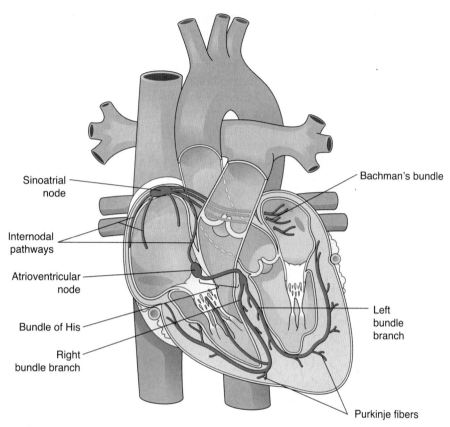

Sinoatrial node

Bachman's bundle

Internodal pathways

Atrioventricular node

Bundle of His

Right bundle branch

Left bundle branch

Purkinje fibers

FIGURE 5-6 Pathway of electrical conduction in the heart. This diagram shows the SA node cells connected to the atrial internodal pathways. In addition, one sees an atrial conduction pathway (called Bachman's bundle) that extends over to the left atrium. Extending into the ventricle from the AV node is the ventricular conduction system, which consists of the bundle of His, the right and left bundle branches, and the Purkinje fibers; these are specialized cardiac muscle cells designed to facilitate rapid distribution of the electrical signal to the ventricles. From McConnell TH. *The Nature of Disease: Pathology for the Health Professions*. Baltimore, MD: Lippincott Williams & Wilkins; 2007.

pass from cell to cell along the specialized conducting pathways (*Figure* 5-6) that travel between both atria (this connection is called Bachman's bundle) and the AV node cells (called the intranodal pathways). The cardiac cells in the conducting pathways have evolved to de-emphasize their contractile function (although they still retain myofibrils) and to emphasize their properties for fast delivery of current from cell to cell; they have a large diameter, and they are connected end to end with many gap junctions. From the conducting pathway, the current passes through gap junctions to the surrounding atrial muscle cells and then, as a wave, from atrial cell to atrial cell, allowing the right and left atrial chambers to contract synchronously. This synchronous contraction allows blood to be pumped from the atria into the ventricles.

Although we have been discussing the need for rapid dissemination of the electrical signal originating in the pacemaker cells to the rest of the heart, we do not want simultaneous contraction of the atria and the ventricles. Simultaneous contraction of all the chambers in the heart would compromise filling of the ventricles and, thus, the amount of blood pumped to the body. Since the ventricles are more muscular chambers than the atria and generate higher pressures during contraction, simultaneous contraction of all the chambers would not permit flow of blood from the atria to the ventricles; contraction of the ventricles leads to closure of the AV valves, thereby preventing flow from atrium to ventricle.

It makes more sense to have the atria contract first into relaxed ventricles, which enables complete ventricular filling. The optimal sequence, therefore, would be atrial contraction, followed by ventricular contraction; this would permit closure of the AV valves *after* the atria have emptied into the ventricles, and subsequent opening of the aortic and pulmonic valves followed by ejection of blood to the lungs and body. For this to occur, there must be a slight delay in the transmission of the electrical signal from the atria to the ventricles.

The two atria are separated from the two ventricles by fibrous connective tissue (the **cardiac skeleton**) in the form of four rings that surround the two atrioventricular orifices as well as the aortic and pulmonary orifices. This band of tissue acts as an electrical insulator, effectively isolating the atria electrically from the ventricles. The only electrically conducting tissue that pierces the cardiac skeleton is an extension beyond the AV node, called the Bundle of His, which is the beginning of the ventricular conduction system (described fully below). In addition, a second mechanism exists to ensure that the atrial and the ventricular chambers have sequential contractions. There is a delay in the speed of conduction of current as it moves through the AV node, prior to transmission of the signal to the bundle of His. The diameter of the cells in the AV node is small, and they have few gap junctions; these factors slow conduction. Taken together, the cardiac skeleton and the structure of the AV node slow the speed of the current as it passes from the atria to the ventricles. This built-in delay allows time for the atria to fully contract before electrical activation moves through the cardiac skeleton and on to the ventricular conducting system.

> **?** **THOUGHT QUESTION 5-1:** **From what you know of the cardiac cycle and the electrical conduction system, what might be the hemodynamic consequence for someone who has a complete block of electrical communication between the atria and the ventricles?**

VENTRICULAR CONDUCTION PATHWAY

Following atrial contraction, the current resulting from action potentials, having passed slowly through the AV node, now enters the ventricular conduction pathway and picks up speed again. The initial segment, called the atrioventricular bundle (or bundle of His), pierces the cardiac skeleton. It then splits into the right and left bundle branches, which run on either side of the interventricular septum; both of these main branches may divide further into many terminal Purkinje fibers. The ventricular conduction pathway functions to distribute the current quickly to the far reaches of the right and left ventricles. From the conducting system, the current passes through gap junctions into the surrounding ventricular muscle cells and then, as a wave, from cell to cell through ventricular muscle, leading to depolarization of individual myocytes, which perpetuates the current and allows the right and left ventricles to contract almost synchronously (left ventricular contraction starts just before that of the right ventricular) to pump blood to the lungs and to the body.

Use Animated Figure 5-5 (Cardiac conduction pathway) to view the sequence of events in depolarization and mechanical activation (contraction) of the heart. Initiate an AP in the SA node and watch as the wave of depolarization propagates, first through the atria, and then, after a delay at the AV node, through the ventricles. Pay particular attention to the coordination between electrical and mechanical events. You can observe how the delay at the AV node allows for ventricular filling, and how the electrical activation of the ventricles initiates (and hence precedes) their mechanical activation (contraction).

Hierarchy of Depolarization—Setting the Heart Rate

All cells within the conduction pathway (SA node, AV node, bundle of His, bundle branches, and Purkinje fibers) are capable of generating spontaneous APs. Why then isn't there electrical chaos with cells each firing independent APs? There is a strict hierarchy in the rate of spontaneous depolarization as you move from proximal portions of the conducting system (starting at the SA node) to distal (ending in the Purkinje fibers) along the conduction system. The key to the hierarchy lies in the slope of spontaneous depolarization during phase 4 of the pacemaker cell AP (*Figure* 5-3). The slope of this segment is steepest in the SA node cells, which means that under normal conditions SA node cells fire an AP before other cells. The electrical impulses then travel along the conduction system, depolarizing all other cells in the pathway before they have a chance to depolarize spontaneously. In this way, the SA node determines the heart rate.

In the event that the SA node cells are dysfunctional and fail to initiate APs, the AV node cells (with the next steepest phase 4 slope) will trigger their own APs. It is important to recognize, however, that because of the lower slope of phase 4 in the AV node cells, it takes longer for these cells to reach threshold and generate an AP; thus, their inherent rate of self depolarization is slower than SA node cells, which results in a slower heart rate. If neither SA node nor AV node cells initiate APs, the bundle branches or Purkinje fibers can take up the job. But you must remember that each time you move more distally down the conducting pathway, the inherent rate of spontaneous depolarization slows. SA nodal rhythm is approximately 70 beats/min, AV nodal rhythm is 40 to 50 beats/min, and Purkinje cell rhythm is about 20 to 30 beats/min. A person who is relying on APs generated in the His–Purkinje system would have a very slow heart rate (and a low cardiac output since cardiac output is the product of heart rate and stroke volume) and, thus, would require an artificial pacemaker.

Animated Figure 5-6 (Backup pacemakers) lets you view the mechanisms that allow the SA node to act as the principal pacemaker under normal circumstances. Notice how, when firing normally, the depolarization initiated by the SA node reaches the other potential pacemakers before they spontaneously reach their threshold potentials. Now knock out any of the pacemaker sites in the figure and watch as the fastest (i.e., highest frequency) remaining pacemaker site takes over. You can see how the difference in the rate of spontaneous depolarization (slope of phase 4) for each of the pacemaker sites allows time for the depolarization initiated by the fastest pacemaker to reach more distal pacemakers before they can fire spontaneously.

> **?** **THOUGHT QUESTION 5-2:** In the example above (Thought Question 5-1), can you now predict (and explain) what the heart rate would be for someone with a complete block between the atrial and the ventricular electrical conduction systems?

Autonomic Influence on Cardiac Electrical System

As stated earlier in the chapter, the pacemaker cells have automaticity and can generate action potentials independently of external controls. For this reason, a denervated heart will still beat, an important characteristic that makes it possible to transplant a heart from one person to another. It is important to remember, however, that changes in autonomic activity (either sympathetic or parasympathetic) have a powerful effect on the rate of spontaneous depolarization of the pacemaker cells, and hence the heart rate.

Panel A

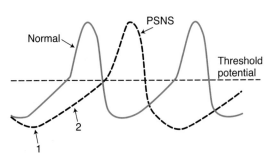

Panel B

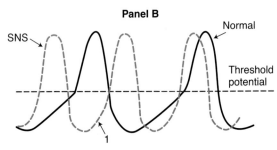

FIGURE 5-7 Effect of stimulation of the autonomic nervous system on pacemaker action potential. Panel A shows two of the three changes made by parasympathetic nervous system (PSNS) activity on the pacemaker action potential: (1) resting membrane potential is more negative, (2) slope of phase 4 depolarization is made less steep, and (3) (not shown) threshold potential is more positive. Panel B shows the change made by sympathetic nervous system (SNS) activity on the pacemaker action potential: (1) the slope of phase 4 depolarization is made steeper.

Stimulation of the parasympathetic nervous system (PSNS) releases acetylcholine, which acts on muscarinic receptors on SA node pacemaker cells and has three effects (Panel A, *Figure* 5-7). Because of alterations in I_f, the slope of phase 4 depolarization is decreased (or flattened), the threshold potential is made more positive (thus, it takes more time to move from the resting to threshold potential), and the starting or resting membrane potential is made more negative (the difference between resting and threshold potentials is greater). Together all these changes slow down the rate of AP generation within the SA node and, thus, the heart rate.

In contrast, increased sympathetic nervous system (SNS) activity releases norepinephrine and epinephrine, which act on adrenergic receptors on SA node pacemaker cells. Again, as a consequence of alterations in I_f, albeit in the opposite direction of the changes resulting from cholinergic effects, the slope of phase 4 depolarization is increased (*Figure* 5-7). This allows the pacemaker cells to reach threshold more quickly and generate action potentials even faster than dictated by their inherent physiology, thereby achieving a higher heart rate.

 Animated *Figure* 5-7 (Effect of ANS on heart rate) illustrates the changes described above. Activate either the SNS or the PSNS and notice the effects on the slope of depolarization, the threshold potential, the starting membrane potential (most negative baseline), and the subsequent effects on the heart rate.

PUTTING IT TOGETHER

You are shadowing a cardiologist when Mr. Luigi Vidello comes in, having been referred by his general practitioner. Mr. Vidello is a fit, athletic 47-year-old man who has noticed increasing fatigue and inability to train in his masters-level soccer league. Several times in the last 6 months he has had to stop mid game to catch his breath, and these episodes have been accompanied by a sensation of lightheadedness. During one of these events he lay down and

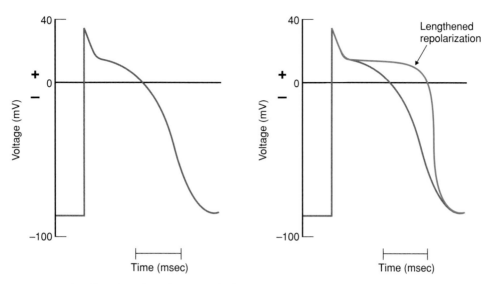

FIGURE 5-8 Normal and lengthened repolarization. This figure shows both a normal cardiac action potential (left panel) and one with a lengthened repolarization phase (right panel), as experienced by the patient, Luigi Vidello.

may have passed out very briefly. His father died suddenly in his early 40s of something related to his heart (he was not sure of the details). His doctor obtained an electrocardiogram (or ECG) and said he found evidence of abnormal repolarization in his ventricles (we will review the principles of the ECG in Chapter 6). At rest in the cardiologist's office, Mr. Vidello's pulse is regular and slow, and his blood pressure is normal. Further analysis of his ECG reveals that his ventricular muscle cells have a delayed, *or lengthened, repolarization period (this relates to phase 3 of the cardiac action potential; Figure 5-8). What might be causing Mr. Vidello's symptoms?*

The primary ion involved with <u>repolarization</u> *is potassium, and its site of entry and exit into the cells is through various voltage-gated potassium channels. Ion channel dysfunctions, called* **channelopathies,** *can run in families. Given Mr. Vidello's family history of sudden cardiac death, there might be reason to suspect he is carrying a gene for a specific potassium channel abnormality. Repolarization abnormalities, such as lengthening of the duration of the action potential, can put the patient at risk of developing serious ventricular rhythm disturbances. During the "relative refractory phase," alterations in potassium channel function can be associated with oscillations in the membrane potential, called "early after-depolarizations," which can lead to very fast heart rates and sudden cardiac death.*

In patients with repolarization abnormalities, the development of serious rhythm disorders (e.g., ventricular fibrillation) are often associated with states of high sympathetic nervous activity, as would be associated with Mr. Vidello's exercise. Treatment for him (among other things) would include prescribing a drug that decreased sympathetic activity or blocked the effects of the sympathetic nervous system on the heart. Finally Mr. Vidello would likely receive an implantable artificial defibrillator, a device that monitors the heart rhythm and, in the event of detection of a dangerously fast or irregular rhythm, administers an electrical shock to return the patient's heart back to a normal electrical function.

Summary Points

- The concentration gradient of ions inside the cell relative to outside the cell and the resulting electrical driving force, which is created when a charged ion enters or exits the cell, determine ion movement into and out of the myocyte.

- Depolarization in an atrial or ventricular cell represents a shift in membrane potential from the cell's initial negative potential (close to the Nernst equilibrium potential for potassium) to a strongly positive potential (close to the Nernst equilibrium potential for sodium).
- In comparison to atrial and ventricular myocytes, depolarization in pacemaker cells starts from a membrane potential that is slightly less negative and goes to a positive potential that is close to the Nernst equilibrium potential for calcium rather than sodium.
- Stage 4 of the action potential in pacemaker cells has an "upward slope" indicative of an ion leak necessary to achieve spontaneous depolarization.
- Repolarization in all cardiac cells (atrial, ventricular, and pacemaker) represents a return from positive to negative membrane potentials, largely as a result of potassium exiting the cell through various potassium channels.
- Action potential (AP) is the term used to describe the sequence of events that characterizes the depolarization and repolarization of a cell.
- There are two types of cardiac muscle cells: (a) those that spontaneously depolarize and initiate their own AP, called pacemaker cells, and (b) those that are activated by the current resulting from the AP passing through gap junctions from an adjacent cardiac cell. Atrial and ventricular cardiac muscle cells are in the second category.
- Pacemaker cells are clustered in two places, called nodes, in the wall of the right atrium. The first cluster is called the sinoatrial (SA) node and the second cluster is called the atrioventricular (AV) node.
- Features unique to pacemaker cell action potentials are a sloped phase 4 (indicative of spontaneous slow depolarization) and a sloped phase 0 upstroke (reflecting the influx of calcium during the rapid phase of depolarization).
- Features unique to ventricular or atrial cell action potentials are a stable resting membrane potential, reflected in a flat phase 4, a sharp, fast phase 0 upstroke (reflecting the influx of sodium during the rapid phase of depolarization), and a plateau called phase 3.
- The absolute refractory period of an action potential spans phases 0, 1, 2 and the initial part of phase 3. During the refractory period, the fast sodium channels remain in their inactivated state and, thus, cannot be recruited for another AP.
- The duration of the absolute refractory period for cardiac cells and the duration of the muscle twitch of the myocytes are very similar. This prevents the heart from undergoing tetanic contractions from repetitive electrical stimulation.
- The atrial conduction pathway comprises the SA node, the intra-atrial pathways, Bachman's bundle, and the AV node. The ventricular conduction pathway comprises the bundle of His, the right and left bundle branches, and the Purkinje fibers.
- The rate of spontaneous depolarization diminishes as one proceeds down the electrical conduction system from atria to ventricles; hence, heart rates driven by action potentials initiated from lower down in the conduction system are slower than those driven by the SA node.
- A band of fibrous tissue (the cardiac skeleton) separates the atria and ventricles; the tissue conducts electricity poorly, thereby preventing general dissemination to the ventricles of current resulting from atrial myocyte APs.
- Coordinated contraction of the upper and lower chambers of the heart is ensured by the inherent controls of the cardiac conduction system.

Answers TO THOUGHT QUESTIONS

5-1.   This condition is called complete heart block, and it describes a situation in which the atrial and the ventricular conducting pathways are operating independently. Under this condition, it is possible that the atria will be depolarized and contract at the same time as the ventricles. In other words, the atria may be contracting against atrioventricular valves that are closed because of simultaneous ventricular contraction. The hemodynamic consequence of complete heart block is that the ventricles are deprived of the relatively small additional volume (at rest) that is contributed by atrial contraction. During activity, however, and in pathologic states in which the LV is very stiff (has low compliance), the contribution to ventricular filling made by atrial contraction becomes more important and, thus, its absence is more of an issue. You might also be asking yourself, what happens to the volume of blood in the atria when they contract against closed valves? Remember that there are no valves between the atria and the large veins returning to the heart. If we use the right side of the heart as an example, atrial contraction against a closed tricuspid valve produces a pressure wave seen as a bounding pulse (called a "cannon a wave") backward into the jugular vein in the neck.

5-2.   In a person with complete heart block, the sinus node is normal and would be initiating a rhythm at its inherent rate of spontaneous depolarization (around 60–100 times/min). Hence, the atria would be contracting at that rate. With block of the electrical communication that normally allows current to flow to the AV node, however, the cells in the AV node (or possibly lower in the ventricular conducting system) are effectively separated from the proximal portion of the cardiac controller. Consequently, there is time for these cells to complete their own spontaneous depolarization and initiate an AP, which ultimately leads to depolarization of the ventricles. If depolarization is occurring at the level of the AV node, whose cells generate APs at a rate of 40 to 50 times a minute, the heart rate would be 40 to 50 beats/min.

Review Questions

1.   Cardiac muscle cells are unable to generate a second action potential <u>during the absolute recovery period</u> for which of the following reasons:

   A.   Calcium channels are open and unable to close
   B.   Fast sodium channels are inactivated and unable to open
   C.   Potassium channels are closed and unable to open
   D.   The funny current is activated

2.   A patient is seen complaining of orthostatic hypotension (as a result of standing up from a lying or sitting position). Two months previously he suffered a myocardial infarction as a result of blockage in his right coronary artery. His resting heart rate is 55 beats/min. When you look at the ECG, you notice that there are no P waves (indicating no coordinated atrial depolarization) and the QRS (indicating ventricular depolarization) waves are normal.
   What is the most likely explanation for his bradycardia?

   A.   Left ventricular damage and low LV ejection fraction as a result of the MI
   B.   Mitral valve insufficiency as a result of the MI
   C.   SA node dysfunction as a result of the MI
   D.   Undiagnosed atrial septal defect independent of the MI

3.   A patient with atrial fibrillation experiences completely chaotic electrical signals throughout the atria accompanied by no coordinated contraction of either atrium. An external electrical shock (called cardioversion) can cause the heart to revert back to sinus rhythm (driven by the SA Node again). A potential danger of the successful cardioversion would be which of the following?

   A.   Cardioversion triggering ventricular fibrillation
   B.   Clots that formed in the quivering atria during fibrillation being pumped to heart or brain
   C.   Profound bradycardia
   D.   Triggering of reentry circuits that produce a tachyarrhythmia

4.   You see a patient at the emergency department who arrives in a state of high anxiety and confusion. His pulse is racing, his skin is hot, his face is red, and he is having trouble seeing. His girlfriend shows you the empty vial of gravol (an anticholinergic) and tells you he swallowed at least 10 pills.
   Which of the following explanations account for his <u>cardiac</u> symptoms?

   A.   Interruption of parasympathetic actions on the SA node
   B.   Interruption of sympathetic actions on the SA node
   C.   Stimulation of β-adrenergic receptors on the SA node
   D.   Stimulation of parasympathetic nerves to the AV node

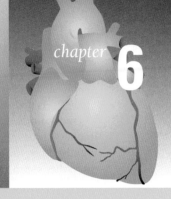

6

Electrocardiogram:
Keeping the Beat

CHAPTER OUTLINE

INTRODUCTION
GENESIS OF THE ELECTROCARDIOGRAM (ECG)
- Einthoven's Triangle and Lead Placement
- Normal ECG Waves and Intervals
- Repolarization and the T Wave
SINGLE-LEAD ECG INTERPRETATION
PHYSIOLOGICAL RHYTHMS

THE ECG AND THE MECHANICAL ACTION OF
 THE CARDIAC PUMP
VENTRICULAR MEAN ELECTRICAL AXIS
- The Normal Axis
- Axis Deviations
PUTTING IT TOGETHER
SUMMARY POINTS

LEARNING OBJECTIVES

By the end of the chapter you will be able to:
- **Explain the following:**
  - **Electrocardiogram (ECG) Lead placement (Einthoven's triangle)**
  - **How the action potential gives rise to the ECG**
  - **Normal ECG waves (P, QRS, T) and intervals (PR, QRS and QT).**
- **Apply basic ECG interpretation skills.**
- **Identify, from single lead samples: normal sinus rhythm, sinus bradycardia, and sinus tachycardia.**
- **Describe the relationship between electrical function and mechanical function of the cardiac chambers.**
- **Describe the significance of the ventricular mean electrical axis.**

Introduction

A solid grasp of the electrical functioning of the heart, as described in Chapter 5, is central to understanding the genesis (and interpretation) of the electrocardiogram or ECG. From your first week in medical school you are likely to be asked by friends and family to interpret an ECG. Remember that sophisticated diagnostic interpretation of ECGs is the focus of a multiyear residency in internal medicine and fellowship in cardiology. Having said that, however, we believe that basic interpretation of ECGs is easily within your grasp during medical school. The first steps of this journey require you to gain an understanding of the principles governing the acquisition of the ECG signal, as well as to learn an approach to deciphering the electrical waves by linking them to a firm understanding of the physiological concepts on which they are based. Developing an approach to ECG interpretation is the first step to making a diagnosis using the ECG.

Under normal conditions, the heart beats in a rhythm called "normal sinus," which implies a heart rate between 60 and 100 beats/min and normal conduction of the electrical impulse from the sinoatrial (SA) node throughout the heart. Various conditions, however, can either speed up or slow down the heart rate, and many disease states can produce disordered or irregular rhythms called arrhythmias. The ECG is a powerful diagnostic tool that is noninvasive, inexpensive, and can provide useful information about the health of a patient.

Genesis of the Electrocardiogram (ECG)

To begin our discussion of the ECG, let us quickly review some of the important electrical principles of the cardiac controller. Under normal conditions, the action potentials (APs) initiated in the SA node create current that triggers additional APs in adjacent cells and current that travels quickly through the atrial conducting pathways, and then from cell to cell throughout the atria. The right and left atria contract synchronously, pumping blood into the ventricles. After a brief delay, the electrical current, which was slowed as it arrived at the atrioventricular (AV) node, then moves rapidly through the ventricular conducting pathways and from there, moves from cell to cell, as each generates its own AP, throughout the ventricular muscle. This process results in near-synchronous contraction of the ventricles, thereby pumping blood to the lungs and the body. The generation of these APs throughout the atrial and ventricular myocytes creates electrical signals. The standard ECG therefore is simply a graphical representation of the summation of millions of electric signals generated by the individual cardiac cells as they depolarize and repolarize.

EINTHOVEN'S TRIANGLE AND LEAD PLACEMENT

To understand the ECG you must first translate the movement of the APs across the heart into what we measure as an ECG. Each AP generates a small electrical signal that triggers an AP in an adjacent cell; the net effect is a "wave" of APs and a small electrical current. The electrical field has both a magnitude and direction. This small, changing electrical field can be amplified and detected by recording electrodes placed on the surface of the body. William Einthoven, a Dutch physician and physiologist at the beginning of the 20th century, although not the first to measure the electrical activity of the heart, was the first person to place recording electrodes in standardized positions on the skin (called leads, see below) for clinical purposes and produced a physical record that he called the Electro**kardio**gram (kardio = heart in Greek) or EKG. In North America, this measurement is referred to as an electro**cardio**gram or ECG, but you may still hear it called an EKG.

With measurements limited to the surface of the body, there is no simple way to assess the wave of electrical activity as it passes from the SA node to the rest of the heart. By using multiple sensors, however, we can assess the magnitude and direction of the electrical impulse in different planes, that is, the component vectors of the impulse. By analogy, imagine tracking the flight of a baseball thrown from second base to first base. You can measure its speed and direction laterally between the bases (one component vector) and its speed vertically (a second component vector). By combining the two vectors, you can get a truer picture of the speed and direction of the baseball at any moment during its flight. Similarly, each ECG lead is basically measuring the component of the electrical impulse in a particular direction. With the information from multiple leads, we can follow the magnitude and direction of the electrical impulse as it travels through the heart, as well as derive the average (net) direction of the electrical impulse (more on this last point when we discuss mean ventricular axis later in the chapter).

Bipolar Limb Leads

A "bipolar limb lead" measures the potential difference between two recording electrodes, one assigned as positive and the other as negative. Einthoven was very particular about where on the body he placed his recording electrodes. In the end, the electrodes formed a virtual triangle, which was eventually named after him (Einthoven's triangle), around the heart (*Figure* 6-1). He put one electrode on the right shoulder (called RA for right arm), one on the left shoulder (called LA for left arm), and one on the abdomen slightly above the left leg (called LL for left leg). Lead I compared the potential difference between the recording electrodes on the RA and the LA, and he designated the LA to be positive and the RA to be negative. Not satisfied with just one "electrical perspective," lead II compared the RA and the LL, with the RA negative and the LL positive. Still not finished, lead III compared the potential difference between the LA and the LL with the LL positive and the LA negative. These leads are simply three different "electrical pictures" of the same heart, each taken from a different perspective, providing a measurement of different component vectors of the impulse. A fourth recording electrode is placed on the abdomen just above the right leg; this is used as a ground electrode and, thus, is not included as part of Einthoven's triangle.

Unipolar Limb Leads

In addition to the bipolar limb leads, we now use three additional leads, called unipolar leads, or augmented limb leads, to assess more completely the electrical impulse in the

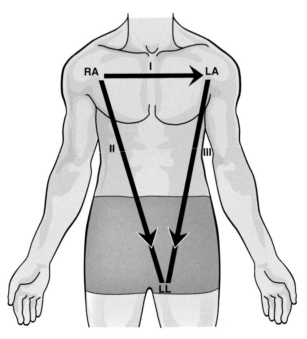

FIGURE 6-1 Einthoven's triangle: This image shows a person with three recording electrodes placed on the chest and trunk and labeled left arm (LA), right arm (RA), and left leg (LL). Bipolar limb leads are formed by comparing the potential difference between any two recording electrodes. Lead I compares the LA to the RA, lead II compares the LL to the RA, and lead III compares the LA to the LL. These three comparisons (or leads) form a triangle around the heart that was named after Willem Einthoven, the father of electrocardiography.

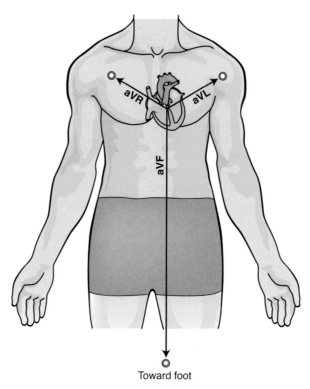

Toward foot

FIGURE 6-2 Augmented limb leads. This image shows three additional limb leads (unipolar leads). The positive end of lead aVR is the right shoulder, the positive end of lead aVL is the left shoulder, and the positive end of aVF is toward the foot (hence the "F" in avF.)

frontal plane. These leads make use of the same electrodes shown in *Figure* 6-1. Instead of being bipolar (one positive end and one negative end), these leads, however, are unipolar, which means that one end is positive, whereas a combination of electrodes (summed together) acts as the negative reference lead (*Figure* 6-2). The first of these unipolar leads is called aVL; the positive end of the lead is the LA. The axis of this lead is a line from left shoulder (positive) to the heart (negative). The second unipolar lead is aVR; the positive end of the lead is RA. The axis of this lead is a line from the right shoulder (positive) to the heart (negative). The third unipolar lead is aVF; the positive end of the lead is the left leg. The axis of this lead is a line from the left leg (positive) to the heart (negative). Together, the bipolar limb leads and the unipolar leads all measure electrical activity in the frontal plane of the body.

Unipolar Chest Leads

Since the heart is a three-dimensional structure, Einthoven also wanted to examine its electrical activity from the perspective of the horizontal plane (*Figure* 6-3). To do that, he needed to add recording electrodes on the surface of the chest moving from the anterior surface (V1 and V2) around the chest (V3 and V4) toward the mid-axillary line (V5 and V6). These recording electrodes form the basis for the "chest" or precordial leads. The six precordial leads are also unipolar; the positive end is represented by each individual recording electrode on the surface of the chest, compared to the single reference lead at zero potential (as described for the unipolar leads). The important difference between the chest leads and the limb leads is that the chest leads are measuring changes in electrical potential in the horizontal plane.

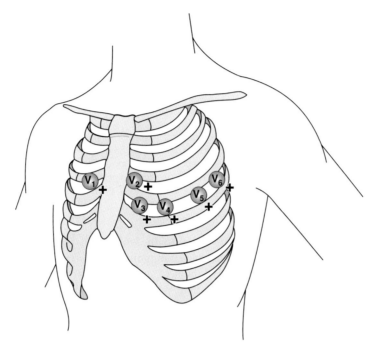

FIGURE 6-3 Shows the six unipolar chest leads (V1 through V6), which measure the electrical activity as it moves through the horizontal plane. (*LifeART* image © Lippincott Williams & Wilkins, 2010. All rights reserved.)

The 12 leads just described allow the practitioner to see a more complete picture of the electrical activity of the heart and represent the standard technique used in the initial approach to clinical diagnosis of cardiac disease. At any point in time, there is a net electrical vector representing the electrical activity of the heart. The ECG is the projection of that vector onto each of the axes or leads of the electrocardiogram. If there is damage or hypertrophy of the myocardium or the conduction system is abnormal, these different electrical perspectives enable the clinician to localize and understand the nature of the problem. Nevertheless, as you will see below, clinically important information with respect to the rhythm of the heart can also be obtained by looking at single-lead ECGs.

NORMAL ECG WAVES AND INTERVALS

Having described the placement of the electrodes, we need to link the electrical activity in the heart to the genesis of an ECG. For simplicity, we will deal initially only with the state of depolarization and we will discuss repolarization later. From this point onward remember that we are dealing with a wave of depolarization (the sum of the millions of electrical fields we mentioned earlier in the chapter). As this depolarization wave moves across the heart and is detected by the recording electrodes, a positive (upward) or negative (downward) pen deflection is recorded on the ECG. Movement of the wave of depolarization toward the positive end of the lead of interest results in an upward ECG pen deflection, and movement toward the negative end of the lead results in a downward ECG pen deflection. When no depolarization is taking place or the depolarization is at right angles to the line between the positive and negative ends of the lead, the ECG pen does not move from its initial position and makes a line called the isoelectric line (*Figure* 6-4). Essentially then, the ECG tracing is a series of up and down pen deflections, the shape of which differs depending on the lead with which you are making the measurement. The maximum

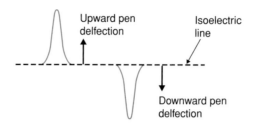

FIGURE 6-4 Up and down pen deflections. The dashed line is the isoelectric line, which represents a state in which there is no electrical activity (depolarization or repolarization) or in which the direction of the electrical impulse is perpendicular to the axis of the lead. When the wave of depolarization is moving toward the positive end of the lead recording the signal, the ECG pen deflects upward; it returns to isoelectric line after the impulse has passed. In contrast, if the wave of depolarization moves away from the positive end of the lead, the ECG pen deflects downward and then returns to the isoelectric line.

amplitude of the ECG deflection relates to the voltage of the electrical signal, which depends upon the mass of heart muscle undergoing depolarization, the direction of the impulse relative to the positive end of the lead, and the distance between the heart and the surface of the body, for example, a patient with very thick chest wall (obesity), hyperinflated lungs (emphysema), or fluid around the heart (pericardial effusion), may have low voltage on the ECG because the distance between the heart and the surface of the body is increased.

> **THOUGHT QUESTION 6-1:** You are evaluating a patient with a history of high blood pressure for many years. As you will learn in Chapter 7, when the heart must generate high pressures for long periods of time, it adapts to the increased stress in the wall of the ventricle by increasing the number of contractile elements in the myocytes; the ventricular wall thickens (a change to which we refer as *hypertrophy*). What do you predict about the size of the deflection associated with the left ventricle in the ECG of this patient compared to a patient without hypertension? Why?

Now that you know what makes the ECG pen move up or down, we can build an entire ECG (atrial and ventricular depolarization) through one cardiac cycle.

P Wave

As electrical activity is initiated in the SA node and moves through the atrial conduction pathways, relatively little heart muscle is activated. Consequently, there is insufficient electrical activity to be picked up by the recording electrodes; the result is that there is no pen movement (the pen remains on the isoelectric line). It is only when the wave of depolarization is moving from cell to cell throughout the atria that the electrical signal is sufficiently strong for the recording electrodes to detect it. In general, depolarization moves in a direction through both atria from right to left and downward (*Figure* 6-5). Look first at lead II (RA negative to LL positive); depolarization through the atria would be traveling in a direction roughly parallel to the long axis of lead II and toward the positive end of the lead. You would expect, therefore, to see an upward pen deflection (called a P wave) during atrial depolarization in this lead.

Since the direction of atrial depolarization is parallel to lead II, it is fairly easy to see why the P wave is represented by an upward pen deflection. It is not as obvious why the other two frontal leads (I and III) generally also have upward P waves. The direction of the

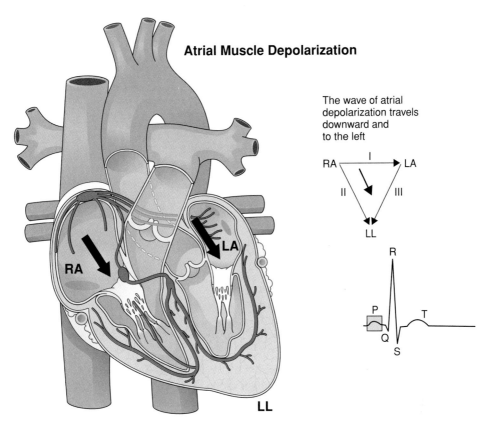

FIGURE 6-5 A P wave is the result of depolarization that travels downward and to the left across both atria (illustrated by two arrows). Consequently, when measuring in lead II (shown in Einthoven's triangle), you would expect to see the P wave as an upward pen deflection. From McConnell TH. *The Nature of Disease: Pathology for the Health Professions*. Baltimore, MD: Lippincott Williams & Wilkins; 2007.

electrical impulse, like a force, can be represented by individual components or vectors at right angles to one another. To help you visualize this, look at *Figure* 6-6. The average direction of the wave of depolarization across the atria is virtually parallel to the long axis of lead II (Panel B) and it is moving toward the positive end; therefore, as we stated above, it will produce a strongly positive or upward pen deflection. Panel A shows that a significant component of the vector represented by atrial depolarization also moves toward the positive end of lead I (although at a more oblique angle to the long axis of the lead), thereby resulting in a weakly positive or smaller upward pen deflection. Panel C illustrates that a component of the vector represented by atrial depolarization is also moving toward the positive end of lead III and similarly produces a small upward pen deflection.

PR Interval

Between the P wave and the QRS wave (below) is a section of the ECG in which the pen returns to and stays on the isoelectric line. The PR interval includes this segment, as well as the P wave. The electrical impulse originating in the SA node is disseminated to the atrial myocytes as well as to the AV node. Because of the fibrous tissue separating the atria from the ventricles, there can be no further movement of the electrical signal directly from atrial to ventricular myocytes. After the atria have depolarized, the electrical signal reflects activity in the cells of the AV node and the conduction pathway just beyond the AV node;

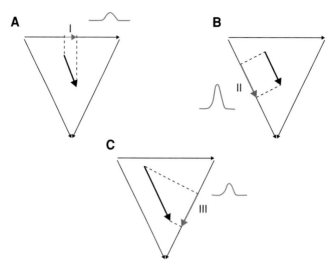

FIGURE 6-6 The three panels show the pen deflection that results from atrial depolarization (moving downward and to the left) in the three frontal leads: I (panel **A**), II (panel **B**), and III (panel **C**). The black arrow in each panel represents the average vector of depolarization in the atria. The red arrow represents the magnitude and direction of that depolarization as seen by each lead. In each case you can see that, *under normal conditions*, the limb leads shown would register an upward or positive P wave.

this activity is insufficient to be recorded by the ECG, and the result is a return to the iso-electric line. A normal PR interval, which indicates normal passage of the electrical signal from atria to ventricles, is a range of values (0.12–0.20 msec) rather than a single number. Diseases of the heart may be associated with abnormally short or long PR intervals. Despite its name, the PR interval is measured on the ECG from the beginning of the P wave until the first deflection away from the isoelectric line after the P wave, whether that is a Q wave or an R wave.

 THOUGHT QUESTION 6-2: You gave a drug to a patient that slows conduction through the AV node. How would you expect that to change the PR interval on that patients ECG?

QRS Wave

In a normal heart, following transit through the ventricular conduction pathway, there is a relatively common pattern to the direction of cell-to-cell depolarization in the ventricles. The first part of the ventricles that begins to depolarize is the interventricular septum; the wave of depolarization goes from left to right. In some leads this is registered as small downward wave, called a Q wave (*Figure* 6-7). Other limb leads do not actually register this wave; in these leads ventricular depolarization starts with a strong upward pen deflection (called an R wave), which represents the wave of depolarization shifting from the interventricular septum to the right and left ventricle. Often, the last part of the ventricles to depolarize is the posterior portion of the muscular left ventricle, which means a wave of depolarization moving toward the posterior and slightly up toward the left shoulder. In some leads that reinforces the strong upward pen deflection (the R wave) and in others it is seen as a large downward deflection (called an S wave). To summarize, ventricular depolarization (relative to atrial depolarization) follows a more complex path, resulting in recordings on the ECG of both upward and downward pen deflections (slightly different in each lead). The three waveforms that commonly make up ventricular

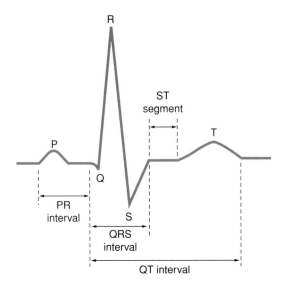

FIGURE 6-7 The ECG waveforms. This figure shows the P, QRS, and T waves and the intervals that are used clinically (the figure is representative of a typical lead I tracing). The Q wave is the first downward wave following a P wave. The R wave is the first upward wave following the P wave. The S wave is the first downward wave following an R wave. Also shown are clinically significant intervals (PR, QRS, QT) and one isoelectric line called the ST segment; this connects the end of the S wave and the beginning of the T wave. To distinguish an interval from a segment, intervals include at least one waveform. Adapted from Smeltzer SC and Bare BG. *Brunner & Suddarth's Textbook of Medical-Surgical Nursing.* 9th ed. Philadelphia, PA: Lippincott Williams & Wilkins, 2000.

depolarization are a downward facing Q wave, followed by an upward facing R wave, followed by a downward facing S wave. Not all of these are necessarily present in any one lead. Under normal conditions, the total duration of these three waves (QRS) should not exceed 0.12 msec.

> **? THOUGHT QUESTION 6-3: A patient has a heart attack that results in slowing of the electrical depolarization throughout the ventricles. How would you expect that to change the QRS wave in this patient's ECG? Why?**

REPOLARIZATION AND THE T WAVE

As you recall from Chapter 5, after cardiac cells depolarize, they repolarize to prepare for the next AP. The ECG machine records the wave of repolarization using the same principle as depolarization. Since repolarization reflects movement of ions in the opposite direction (positive ions leaving the cells) of what is seen with depolarization (positive ions coming into the cell), the direction of the pen deflections is a bit more complicated. One must consider both the direction of the electrical impulse (toward or away from the positive lead) as well as the direction of the ion movement. For example, when a wave of **repolarization** moves toward the positive end of the lead, the pen deflects downward, not upward as in depolarization, because of the opposite direction of ion movement (*Figure 6-8*).

That being the case, you might think that the waveform on the ECG that represents ventricular depolarization (QRS wave) would be in the opposite direction to ventricular repolarization (T wave). That would be true if *depolarization and repolarization occurred in the same direction.* In human hearts, however, the last cells to depolarize are the first to repolarize; the wave of repolarization occurs *in the opposite direction* to depolarization and,

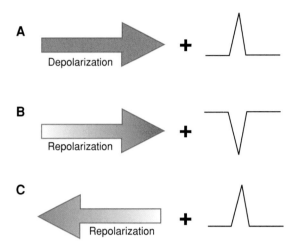

FIGURE 6-8 Depolarization and repolarization. During depolarization, a positive deflection is seen if the direction of the electrical impulse (shown by the arrow) is toward the positive end of the lead (**A** above). During repolarization, the cell is going from a positive to a negative charge (opposite what occurs during depolarization); the direction *of the ECG deflection*, therefore, will be opposite what is seen for any given lead during depolarization as long as the path of repolarization is traveling in the same direction as the depolarization (**B**). When a wave of repolarization travels in the opposite direction as depolarization (as happens in the heart and shown in **C**), the pen deflection is the same as the initial depolarization (**A** and **C**). For example, the QRS deflection, signifying depolarization of the ventricle, is upright in lead I. The T wave, signifying repolarization of the ventricle, is also upright in lead I.

therefore, produces *a pen deflection* that goes in the same direction as depolarization (the direction of the electrical signal is opposite of what occurs during depolarization, and the direction of ion movement is opposite of depolarization; in a sense, two "negatives" make a "positive"). This concept can be tricky the first time through, but it is an important one, so take the time to work it out before you move on.

The waveform that represents ventricular repolarization is called the T wave. The pathway of repolarization of the ventricles is less complex than the pathway for depolarization, and it does not travel through the specialized conduction system as does depolarization; the result is a shallower and wider waveform on the ECG. Therefore, the T wave is generally a relatively simple waveform compared to the QRS, which represents ventricular depolarization.

Animated Figure 6-1 (Cardiac conduction and ECG waves) illustrates the correspondence of the P, QRS, and T waves, as well as the PR interval, to the cardiac conduction pathway and atrial and ventricular depolarization. First, play the overall sequence to get a real-time idea of how the rapid conduction phase, depolarization of atrial and ventricular muscle cells, and contraction are temporally and spatially related. Then step through the diagram slowly and observe the correspondence between the ECG waves (P, QRS, and T) and the progression of cardiac depolarization. You can also use the diagram to follow along with the discussion in the previous pages.

? THOUGHT QUESTION 6-4: In the description of the ECG, we have discussed the P wave (atrial depolarization), the QRS complex (ventricular depolarization), and the T wave (ventricular repolarization). Where on the ECG is atrial repolarization?

? THOUGHT QUESTION 6-5: If you were assessing the heart using lead aVR, would you expect atrial depolarization to be recorded as an upward or downward P wave? Why?

TABLE 6-1 APPROACH TO SINGLE LEAD ECG INTERPRETATION
1. Establish the rate
2. Establish the rhythm
3. Identify the P waves
4. Measure the PR interval
5. Measure the width of the QRS complex

This table illustrates an approach to ECG interpretation whereby you methodically examine each item (1–5) in sequence: rate, rhythm, P waves, the duration of the PR interval, and, finally, the duration of the QRS complex. Ultimately, you will also need to assess the segments (PR, ST) and waveforms (particularly the T wave) that may change with various pathologic conditions.

Single-Lead ECG Interpretation

When you are just beginning to learn about ECGs, a good place to start is by reviewing what is called a "single-lead ECG." These ECGs are recorded on one lead (often one of the three limb leads: I, II, or III). Everything we have discussed in this chapter thus far applies to looking at single-lead ECGs. When looking at an ECG, it is important to have a systematic approach to your analysis. One approach is shown in Table 6-1.

Initially, you look at the rate and ask yourself the following questions: Is it within the normal range (60–100 beats/min at rest)? Is it fast (tachycardia > 100 beats/min at rest) or slow (bradycardia < 60 beats/min at rest)? Next, you look at rhythm and ask yourself: Is it regular (consistent R-R interval), irregular with a pattern (e.g., beat-beat-pause, beat-beat-pause), or irregular with no pattern (e.g., beat-pause, beat-beat-pause, beat-pause-beat-beat-beat)? Third, you look at the P waves and analyze whether they are present (i.e., identifiable as P waves), are of the same shape, and whether they all are associated with a QRS complex (each P is followed by a QRS, every QRS is preceded by a P wave). Fourth, you look at the PR interval. This is measured from the beginning of the P wave to the initiation of the R wave and relates to atrial depolarization and the delay at the AV node. Again, you assess whether the PR interval is within the normal range (0.12–0.20 sec), or is abnormally long (>0.20 sec) or short (<0.12 sec). If it is longer, you must look to see if the interval is consistently longer (i.e., unchanging) or whether the interval is increasing in length with each consecutive beat. These distinctions in PR interval can have important implications in determining several important arrhythmias. Finally, you measure the width of the QRS wave. You determine whether the duration is within the normal range (<0.12 sec), or wider than normal (>0.12 sec). An abnormally wide QRS complex may imply that electrical conduction is not accessing the normal ventricular conduction pathway; rather, it may be traveling slowly through ventricular muscle, thereby prolonging depolarization and widening the QRS complex. There are many different approaches to the interpretation of ECGs; which one you select is less important than **that you select one** and use it routinely.

Physiological Rhythms

Now that you have a feel for how the ECG is generated, there are three rhythms that you need to recognize in normal cardiac physiology: normal sinus rhythm, sinus bradycardia, and sinus tachycardia.

Normal Sinus Rhythm (NSR) describes a healthy electrical conduction system. The SA node is initiating APs, which then access the normal atrial and ventricular conducting pathways (normal P, QRS, and T waves), leading to a heart rate within the range of 60 to 100 beats/min. *Figure* 6-9, panel A, is an example of a single-lead ECG showing an NSR. In this figure, you can see the P waves are present, they are all similar in shape, and they face

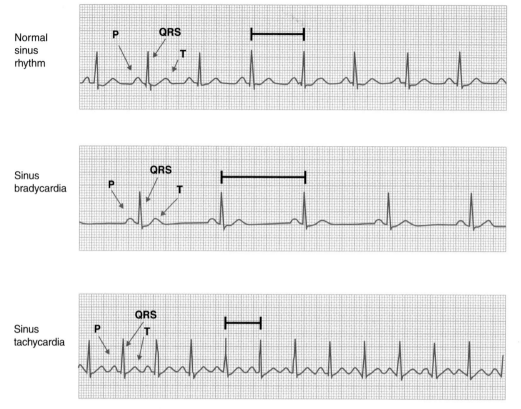

FIGURE 6-9 These ECG strips are all representative of physiological rhythms: top panel is normal sinus rhythm, middle panel is sinus bradycardia, and bottom panel is sinus tachycardia.

in the same direction; the observation that they are all the same shape and direction indicates that the P waves have the same site of origin within the heart. In addition, every P wave is associated with a QRS wave, which suggests that ventricular activation is due to conduction of the electrical signal from the atria to the ventricles.

Sinus bradycardia (*Figure* 6-9; panel B) is similar to NSR but the heart rate is slower (<60 beats/min). In this rhythm, P waves are present, similar in shape, all facing the same direction (all upward deflections), and each P wave gives rise to a QRS wave; the heart rate, however, is less than 60 beats/min.

Sinus tachycardia (*Figure* 6-9; panel C) is similar to NSR but the heart rate is faster than normal (>100 beats/min). In this rhythm, P waves are present, similar in shape, all facing the same direction (all upward deflection), and each P wave gives rise to a QRS wave; the heart rate, however, is greater than 100 beats/min. Normal physiological conditions associated with increased sympathetic nervous system activity, such as exercise, are characterized by sinus tachycardia.

The ECG and the Mechanical Action of the Cardiac Pump

The electrical activity of the heart is designed to produce coordinated synchronous contraction and relaxation of the chambers. For simplicity sake, we will focus on the ventricles, although the process is similar in the atria, and quickly review the relationship between the action potential and contraction (and relaxation) of the myocyte.

In order to achieve contraction of the ventricular muscle, all the individual cells must undergo a series of ionic shifts—the rapid upstroke (phase 0) of the cardiac AP (associated with sodium influx), followed by the opening, during phase 2, of the calcium channels, which are instrumental in **calcium-induced calcium release** within the cells (refer to *Figure* 5-1; also see Animated Figure 3-2 for a review of calcium-induced calcium release). This calcium, released from the intracellular sarcoplasmic reticulum (SR), promotes cross-bridge formation between myosin and actin fibrils and leads to contraction of the myocardial cells. Following depolarization and calcium release, there must be a period of repolarization during which the membrane voltages return to their resting, negative levels. This is phase 3 of the AP, during which potassium leaves the cells and calcium is actively removed from the cross bridges (pumped out of the cell or back into the SR). Removal of calcium from the contractile apparatus results in ventricular relaxation. This process is critical to enable the ventricles to fill prior to the next contraction.

Ventricular Mean Electrical Axis

THE NORMAL AXIS

The standard ECG is a graphical representation of the summation of millions of electric fields generated by the individual cardiac cells as they depolarize and repolarize. If you average the electrical force over the time course of ventricular depolarization, you get a vector called the **ventricular "mean electrical axis"** or ventricular MEA; this can be characterized with respect to its amplitude and direction. Estimating the MEA, which is only measured in the frontal plane, will be important to you as clinicians since an abnormal MEA can point to various pathophysiological conditions. Values of MEA found to be outside the normal range are called axis deviations and can indicate changes in heart position, changes in heart mass, or disturbances in electrical function (more details on axis deviations below).

To estimate ventricular MEA, you need a patient's ECG and something called the hexaxial system of Bayley (HSB). The HSB is created by taking all the frontal leads (I, II, III, aVR, aVL, aVF), as they are represented on the body, and bisecting them in the center (*Figure* 6-10). Once compiled, the leads form a circular grid separated by 30° intervals. The positive ends of each lead are labeled in *Figure* 6-10.

Figure 6-11 illustrates how you apply the HSB to an ECG to estimate the ventricular MEA. For this measurement, you need to have at least two leads from the patient's 12-lead ECG. Select two leads whose long axes are at right angles; by convention, leads I and aVF are chosen. Starting with lead I (panel A), examine the QRS complex and observe whether it is more positive (upward) or negative (downward). In this example, it is more positive than negative. Second, you look at the HSB in panel B. Lead I is represented by the solid line. When the QRS in lead I is positive, the vector for depolarization of the ventricles must be projecting somewhere in the right half of the circle, that is, to the right of the perpendicular dotted line. To narrow down the MEA vector's position further, you do the same thing for lead aVF. Look at the QRS (panel C) and observe that it is more positive than negative. Look at the HSB in panel D, with aVF drawn as a solid line. Depolarization must, therefore, be represented by a vector in the bottom half of the circle, that is, below the dotted line. The final step (panel E) is to put the two observations together. The only quadrant from panels B and D that shows overlap and, therefore, represents the common MEA for this patient is the one between 0° to +90°. The MEA, therefore, must be somewhere between those two values. A vector between 0° and 90°, that is, pointing downward and to the left side of the body, represents a normal MEA. When your knowledge about ECGs becomes

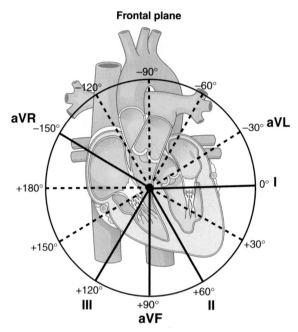

FIGURE 6-10 The hexaxial system of Bayley is a collection of all the frontal leads arranged on paper such that they bisect each other. This creates a configuration in which the long axis of each lead is separated by an angle of 30°. The leads on the top half of the circle go from 0 to −180°, whereas the bottom half go from 0 to +180°. The frontal leads are all marked on the diagram such that they are labeled at the positive end of the lead. From McConnell TH. *The Nature of Disease: Pathology for the Health Professions.* Baltimore, MD: Lippincott Williams & Wilkins; 2007.

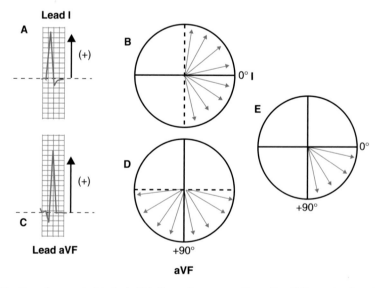

FIGURE 6-11 Estimation of mean electrical axis: This figure shows a mostly positive QRS complex from lead I (panel **A**). Using the hexaxial system of Bayley (panel **B**), the vector representing the ventricular MEA must be to the right of the dashed line, or toward the positive end of lead I. Panel **C** shows a mostly positive QRS complex from lead aVF. Using the hexaxial system of Bayley (panel **D**), you can determine that the vector representing the ventricular MEA must be below the dashed line, or toward the positive end of lead aVF. Putting these two observations together (panel **E**), the overlapping quadrant is between 0° and +90°. This represents a normal MEA, that is, downward and to the left side of the patient.

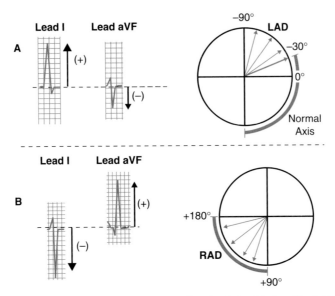

FIGURE 6-12 Axis deviations. Panel A includes QRS complexes from lead I (positive) and lead aVF (negative). The overlapping quadrant, therefore, is between 0° and −90°. The range of normal MEA extends from +90° to −30° (shown in panel **A**). If the vector lies between −30° and −90°, however, it represents a left-axis deviation (LAD). Panel **B** includes QRS complexes from lead I (negative) and lead aVF (positive). The overlapping quadrant, therefore, is between 90° and 180°, and represents a right-axis deviation (RAD).

more sophisticated, you will find that the normal MEA range extends slightly outside the 0° to +90° landmarks (0° to −30° is also within the normal range). By using additional leads (beyond I and aVF), you can pinpoint the MEA with greater specificity.

AXIS DEVIATIONS

If you see an ECG with a positive QRS in lead I coupled with a negative QRS in Lead aVF, it reflects an MEA between 0° and −90°, which is referred to as a left-axis deviation (*Figure 6-12; panel A*). (You may also see left-axis deviation being defined as the region between −30° and −90°.) Alternatively, an ECG with a negative QRS in lead I and a positive QRS in aVF would have an MEA between +90° and +180° or a right-axis deviation (panel B). Axis deviations have many potential explanations, from a simple positional change in the heart (e.g., during pregnancy when the heart is pushed more horizontally) to an increase in ventricular muscle mass (e.g., left ventricular hypertrophy sometimes results in left-axis deviation, and right ventricular hypertrophy often leads to a right-axis deviation). You can see how a simple, noninvasive test such as an ECG can provide vital information about cardiac physiology and pathophysiology.

 Use Animated Figure 6-2 to see how inspection of two perpendicular limb leads (such as I and aVF) allows you to estimate the direction of the mean ventricular axis.

PUTTING IT TOGETHER

You are volunteering in Student Health Services at your university when Paul, a 22-year-old student, is brought in. He is acutely intoxicated and complaining that his heart is "jumping all over the place." He is badly slurring his words and admits to having had "a lot" to drink over the previous 2 hours. He denies taking any drugs. He says he feels light headed intermittently.

Paul's ECG

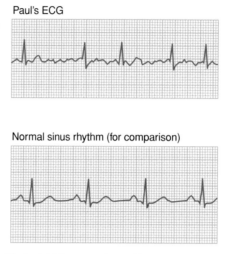

Normal sinus rhythm (for comparison)

FIGURE 6-13 Paul's ECG. Top panel is the ECG from "Paul," and bottom panel is an ECG showing normal sinus rhythm for comparison.

He is tachycardic and his pulse is irregular; his blood pressure is 90/50 mm Hg. The doctor runs a single-lead ECG (Figure 6-13). What cardiovascular factors are contributing to his symptoms, physical examination findings, and ECG?

Several things differentiate Paul's single-lead ECG from one with a NSR. The rate is fast (~100 beats/min), and there are no discernable P waves; rather the baseline, or isoelectric line, is wavy and unstable. Furthermore, the R-to-R interval (distance between two consecutive QRS complexes) is irregular in Paul's ECG compared to the even spacing of the complexes in NSR.

Paul has paroxysmal atrial fibrillation, which may be part of what is called "Holiday Heart" syndrome when it is seen as a consequence of acute alcohol ingestion. In Paul's case, the high level of alcohol in his blood has resulted in disorganization of depolarization and repolarization in both his atria. As a result, his SA node is no longer driving the rhythm of his heart. Instead, his AV node is receiving rapid volleys of electrical signals from APs arising from various directions across his right atrium. Depending on whether or not the AV node cells are refractory at the time they receive an electrical impulse, the APs are either stopped (AV node is refractory) or communicated down the ventricular conducting system (AV node cells not refractory), resulting in a ventricular depolarization and contraction. This process produces an irregular ventricular rhythm with no discernable pattern. This is sometimes referred to as an "irregularly irregular" rhythm.

This rhythm can be dangerous to Paul if it goes untreated. If the ventricular rate is high enough, it can decrease cardiac output (too little time to fill the ventricle) and result in hypotension. In addition, because his atria are no longer performing synchronous contractions (they are quivering not pumping), the absence of coordinated atrial activity deprives the ventricle of the extra filling that occurs at the end of diastole when the atrium normally contracts; the stroke volume is, thereby, reduced. Furthermore, the blood in the quivering atria can become stagnant (absent organized contraction in the atrium, blood may pool), a situation that promotes clot formation. If clots are released into the right ventricle, they can travel to the lungs and result in a pulmonary embolism; if they are released into the left ventricle, they can travel to the brain or the coronary arteries and result in a stroke or myocardial infarction.

Treatment for Paul's alcohol-induced condition is largely supportive. One needs to identify and correct hypovolemia and laboratory abnormalities such as hypoglycemia and hypokalemia. Since alcohol poisoning can alter the respiratory controller as well as the cardiac controller, respiratory rate and oxygenation also need to be monitored. He is watched closely while the alcohol in his system is metabolized by the liver, after which the heart will typically resume an NSR.

Summary Points

- The electrocardiogram is a physical representation of the summed electrical currents that result from cardiac depolarization and repolarization.
- When a wave of depolarization moves toward the positive end of the lead from which you are measuring, the ECG pen deflects upward.
- When a wave of depolarization moves away from the positive end of the lead from which you are measuring, the ECG pen deflects downward.
- There are three categories of ECG leads: bipolar limb leads (I, II, and III), unipolar limb leads (aVR, aVL, aVF), and unipolar chest leads (V1 to V6). Clinically, the unipolar and bipolar limb leads are grouped together as limb leads. The limb leads record electrical potentials in the frontal plane, and the chest leads record electrical potentials in the horizontal plane.
- Ventricular depolarization is represented by the QRS complex. The first downward pen deflection after a P wave is called the Q wave. The first upward pen deflection following a P wave is called the R wave, and the first downward pen deflection after an R wave is called the S wave.
- The current of repolarization in the ventricle is in the opposite direction of depolarization. In addition, the direction of repolarization (the cell is going from positive to negative charge) is opposite to depolarization. To determine the deflection of a repolarization wave relative to depolarization, one must consider both of these factors. For the T wave, which represents repolarization of the ventricle, the deflection is generally in the same direction as the predominant direction of the QRS wave.
- Sinus rhythm implies that the AP is originating in the SA node.
- Sinus bradycardia describes a sinus rhythm with a heart rate under 60 beats/min.
- Sinus tachycardia describes a sinus rhythm with a heart rate over 100 beats/min.
- The vector that describes the average direction and amplitude of ventricular depolarization is called the ventricular MEA. It can be estimated using a 12-lead ECG tracing. Deviations outside the normal range are called left- axis deviation and right-axis deviation and can indicate cardiac pathology.

Answers TO THOUGHT QUESTIONS

6-1. The increased muscle mass associated with hypertrophy of the ventricle leads to a larger voltage when the ventricular cells depolarize. Thus, the deflection of the ECG associated with ventricular depolarization (called the QRS wave—more on this below) will be larger in this patient than in an individual without a history of high blood pressure. This observation can assist you in deciding how long the patient's hypertension has been present, since it takes many months for hypertrophy to develop.

6-2. A drug that slowed the AP as it traveled through the AV node would delay the time interval between atrial depolarization and the onset of ventricular depolarization. On the ECG, that would be manifested as a longer than usual PR interval.

6-3. In a patient who sustained damage to the ventricular conduction system as a result of a heart attack, there would be resultant changes to the ECG. The electrical impulse generated by the AP would no longer be able to traverse the fast ventricular conduction system; consequently, the QRS complex will be widened. Unable to traverse fast-conducting fibers, the electrical impulse will be directed through ventricular myocardium, which is a slower and more circuitous route that results in a wider than normal QRS complex (>120 msec). In addition, the QRS complex could have a different constellation of up and down pen deflections, depending on where in the conduction system the damage occurs.

6-4. Atrial repolarization is rarely seen because it occurs at the same time as the ventricles are depolarizing. Since the ventricles represent a much large proportion of cardiac muscle (and hence greater electrical current and voltage), the QRS waveform masks any pen deflections that would represent atrial repolarization.

6-5. In lead aVR, the positive end of the lead is on the right shoulder and the axis of that lead points upward and to the right (to the positive end of the lead). The atria depolarize from the right heart downward and to the left, in other words away from the positive end of lead aVR. Therefore, you would expect the P wave to be downward, that is, a negative deflection.

Review Questions

1. A patient is diagnosed with something called Wolff-Parkinson-White (WPW) syndrome. This describes the presence of an accessory pathway that allows the electrical signal to travel directly to the ventricular muscles, bypassing the normal route through the AV node and along the ventricular conduction system. Which of the following changes would you expect to see in the ECG?

    A. Abnormal T waves
    B. Irregular rhythm with a pattern
    C. No P waves
    D. Tachycardia
    E. Widening of the QRS complex

2. The ECG below was obtained in an exercise physiology laboratory where an evaluation of an elite level athlete (training for the Tour de France) was taking place.

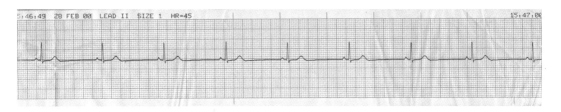

    Which of the following rhythms would best describe his ECG?

    A. Sinus bradycardia
    B. Normal sinus rhythm
    C. Sinus tachycardia

3. A 73-year-old man presents to the Emergency Department complaining of palpitations. His blood pressure 120/80 mm Hg. His single-lead ECG (shown here) would best be described as:

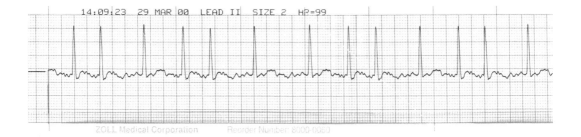

    A. Bradycardic, biphasic P waves, rhythm regular, narrow QRS waves
    B. Bradycardic, no relationship of P waves to QRS, rhythm: irregular with no pattern, narrow QRS waves
    C. Bradycardic, sinus rhythm, rhythm: irregular with a pattern, wide QRS waves
    D. Tachycardic, no discernable P waves, rhythm: irregular with no pattern, narrow QRS waves
    E. Tachycardic, normal P waves, rhythm: regular, wide QRS waves
    F. Tachycardic, sinus rhythm, rhythm: irregular with a pattern, wide QRS waves

4. A 63-year-old female patient with a history of chronic poorly managed pulmonary hypertension has a 12-lead ECG. You look at leads I and aVF. What is the most likely observation you would expect to see?

    A. Large R wave in lead aVF and large S wave in lead I
    B. Large R wave in lead aVF and large R wave in lead I
    C. Large S wave in lead aVF and large R wave in lead I
    D. Same size R and S waves in aVF and large R wave in lead I

5. A 72-year-old male patient suffers a heart attack (myocardial infarction) because of a severe blockage of a branch of the right coronary artery, which supplies the atrioventricular node (AV node) of the heart. You would expect an ECG to show which of the following effects:

    A. Bradycardia
    B. No change in heart rate
    C. Tachycardia
    D. Asystole

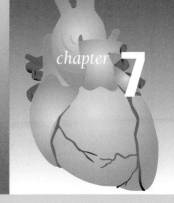

chapter 7

Cardiac Output (Starling Curves):
Getting It Started

CHAPTER OUTLINE

LEARNING OBJECTIVES

By the end of the chapter you will be able to:
• **Describe the determinants of heart rate and stroke volume (autonomic nerves and hormones) in the control of cardiac output.**
• **Delineate the effects of changes in preload (Frank–Starling law), afterload, and contractility on cardiac output, using the ventricular function curve and pressure volume loops.**
• **Describe techniques for measuring cardiac output and ejection fraction.**

Introduction

The most common indicator of the function of the heart is how much blood it pumps out per minute, which is called the cardiac output. The cardiovascular controller, which includes the autonomic nervous system (ANS) and various hormones, plays a major role in increasing or decreasing cardiac output depending on the metabolic needs of the body. The sympathetic limb of the ANS is activated when the body is stressed and leads to an increase in heart rate and stroke volume, both of which augment the output of the heart. In contrast, the parasympathetic limb serves as the braking mechanism, slowing the heart rate and decreasing cardiac output.

In addition to the cardiovascular controller, there are mechanical factors that contribute to cardiac output. The degree to which the ventricle is filled prior to contraction (preload) is one of the determinants of the force that can be generated with contraction (increasing the filling increases the cardiac output); this is referred to as the Frank–Starling law of the heart. The tension or stress in the walls of the heart during systole, called the afterload, is another important determinant of cardiac output; factors that increase afterload, particularly changes in resistance of the blood vessels, tend to decrease the cardiac output. And finally the strength of contraction of the heart (independent of filling), called contractility, which can be altered by changes in the ANS, hormones, and drugs, is another important player in increasing or decreasing cardiac output.

Cardiac Output

HEART RATE AND STROKE VOLUME

In this chapter, we focus on the processes that determine the flow of blood to the body. We start with an examination of factors that influence the volume of blood that arrives on the right side of the heart, and then investigate the determinants of blood flow from the right ventricle to the lungs. From there, we must understand the conditions that alter filling of the left side of the heart and, finally, identify the factors that determine the quantity of blood that is pumped out to the body, that is, the cardiac output.

At its most basic level, cardiac output (CO) is heart rate (HR) multiplied by stroke volume (SV).

$$CO \text{ (mL/min)} = HR \text{ (beats/min)} \times SV \text{ (mL/beat)}$$

In steady-state conditions, the volume of blood that is pumped out of the right heart and that which is pumped out of the left heart are equal; the CO of the right and left ventricles must be the same when averaged over time. On a beat-to-beat level, however, acute changes in contractility or filling of the ventricles (preload) lead to transient inequalities in stroke volume between the ventricles. For example, with inspiration, increased negative intrathoracic pressure transiently increases venous return to the right heart while decreasing venous return to the left heart (remember physiological splitting of S2 from Chapter 4). These inequalities are, however, equalized over time matching cardiac outputs between the right and left ventricles.

The normal CO, when an individual is resting, is about 5 L/min. That may not seem impressive, at first glance. If you multiply that figure over 1 day, however, and then over the average lifespan (80 years), you are now talking about roughly 210,240,000 L. The average 50-m pool contains 1,875,000 L of water, which means that, over an average life span, your heart pumps the volume of approximately 112 Olympic-size swimming pools through your body. And that is assuming a lifetime of resting. If you take into consideration that during exercise the cardiac output can increase up to 5 or 6 times the level at rest . . . well you get the picture.

Stroke volume at rest is 70 mL/beat in the average size person and the resting HR is around 70 beats/min; using the equation above, we get a CO of 4,900 mL/min (or close to 5 L/min). In an average 70-kg male, the total blood volume in the body is ~5 L (4.5 L in a 60-kg female). This means that, at rest, the heart pumps the equivalent of the total blood volume through the body every minute. In a young, healthy person, during maximal exercise, SV can easily double and HR can increase by approximately threefold, which means CO is on the order of 140 mL/beat × 180 beats/min or 25,200 mL/min (~25 L/min, a fivefold to sixfold increase from the resting state).

AUTONOMIC AND HORMONAL CONTROL

The most critical role of the heart is to maintain cardiac output at a level sufficient to satisfy the metabolic needs of the body. Given that requirement, it is important to be able to regulate HR and SV to accommodate the activity of the muscles and the organs.

Control of HR and SV is a critical role of the two limbs of the ANS (sympathetic and parasympathetic).

Regulation of Heart Rate

Let us start with the regulation of HR. We addressed the details of the control of HR in the chapter on the electrical function of the heart (Chapter 5); suffice it to say, if you increase the output of the sympathetic nervous system (SNS), you speed up the HR. The SNS can be thought of as the overdrive mechanism; it speeds up the inherent rhythmicity of the pacemaker cells in the SA node. Conversely, the parasympathetic nervous system (PSNS) acts as the braking mechanism and slows down the HR.

At rest, the heart is predominantly under the influence of the PSNS, that is, it beats more slowly than it would if the parasympathetic nerves were not there. In laboratory studies of animals, for example, if you cut the parasympathetic nerves to the heart, it beats faster. An alternative approach to study this issue is to examine the effects on heart rate of increasing parasympathetic activity. In a study conducted on cardiac surgery patients in whom the cardiac parasympathetic nerves to the heart were stimulated, the researchers were able to drop the HR to 0; the heart stopped completely. When the PSNS is stimulated or a drug is used to reduce the heart rate, we characterize the result as a **negative chronotropic effect** (chrono = time). The three mechanisms behind this effect (review *Figure* 5-5, panel A; and Animated Figure 5-7: Effect of ANS on heart rate) involve the action of acetylcholine on muscarinic receptors found on SA node pacemaker cells: the slope of phase 4 depolarization decreases, the resting membrane potential becomes more negative, and the threshold potential becomes more positive. Together these changes slow the rate at which the threshold for depolarization is achieved and, consequently, slow the heart rate.

Conversely, stimulation of cardiac sympathetic nerves to the heart "revs things up." Both norepinephrine, released from the cardiac sympathetic nerves, and epinephrine, released from the adrenal medulla (with subsequent transport to the heart via the blood stream) have a direct effect on the pacemaker cells in the heart. Norepinephrine and epinephrine increase the slope of phase 4 depolarization, so that the frequency of generation of action potentials in increased, which increases the heart rate (review *Figure* 5-5, panel B; and Animated Figure 5-7: Effect of ANS on heart rate). We refer to this action as a **positive chronotropic** effect. As a result of sympathetic nerve stimulation, HR can triple above its resting level.

Regulation of Stroke Volume (SV)

Let us focus now on regulation of **SV**. Stimulation of heart muscle cells by sympathetic activity increases the strength of contraction. This is called a positive **inotropic effect** (ino = muscle) and, as a result of this effect, SV increases. The mechanism behind this SNS-induced increase in SV is based upon the concept of excitation–contraction (EC) coupling (review Chapter 3).

Stimulation of cardiac sympathetic nerves, and the subsequent release of norepinephrine or epinephrine, produces a positive inotropic action through a β-adrenergic–associated increase in cyclic AMP, which in turn allows more calcium to enter the myocyte. More calcium promotes **cross-bridge cycling** (see Chapter 3) and, thus, a stronger contraction. Cyclic AMP also stimulates protein kinase A; the result is an increase in the intracellular calcium stores and, therefore, increased strength of contraction. A final effect of cyclic AMP is to increase sarcoplasmic reticulum (SR) pump activity, which in turn increases the rate of calcium sequestration in the SR. This action (known as a **lusitropic effect**) shortens the time spent in systole, allows more time in diastole for ventricular filling, and, thereby, increases stroke volume and cardiac output.

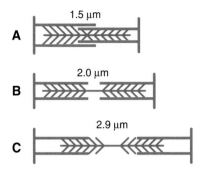

FIGURE 7-1 The length–tension relationship. This figure shows a cartoon depicting three different states of overlap of thick (myosin) and thin (actin) myofibrils at different precontraction sarcomere lengths. Panel **B** shows optimal overlap, and hence optimal cross-bridge formation and tension development, whereas panel **A** shows a short sarcomere length at which the actin fibers just begin to overlap, thereby reducing cross-bridge formation and tension development. Panel **C** shows a long sarcomere length at which cross-bridge formation is again reduced, this time resulting from the stretching apart of the actin filaments.

The Starling Principle. Stroke volume is also controlled by an intrinsic regulatory system of the heart muscle. By "intrinsic," we mean a property of the cardiac muscle itself, independent of nerves and hormones. This feature of cardiac muscle is referred to as the **Frank–Starling law of the heart**. The name of this principle is derived from the two physiologists, Otto Frank and Ernest Starling, who together elaborated the following important concepts.

As you remember from our discussion of EC coupling in Chapter 3, the length of the muscle is positively correlated with the strength of the ultimate contraction. In other words, if you stretch cardiac muscle (within limits) before stimulating it to contract, the tension developed by the muscle is greater than had you not stretched it. We refer to this phenomenon as the **length–tension relationship** (*Figure 7-1*). The observation relies on the fact that the greater the passive stretch, the closer the muscle approaches its optimal amount of overlap of myosin and actin fibrils and, thus, the optimal cross-bridge formation. In cardiac muscle, however, two additional mechanisms contribute to the generation of increased tension with increased length. Increased stretch increases the affinity of troponin for calcium, and it increases the sensitivity of ryanodine receptors to calcium through a mechanism involving nitric oxide. Both of these calcium-related phenomena increase tension generation in cardiac muscle.

Let us translate the length–tension relationship into some workable cardiovascular terms with reference to the heart. To do this, we must make a conceptual jump from an isolated muscle strip generating force in the same direction as contraction to a nearly spherical chamber comprising thousands of muscle cells acting together to generate a force at an angle to the direction of contraction of the individual myocytes.

Between contractions (during diastole), the relaxed ventricles fill with blood. The walls of the chambers stretch to accommodate the incoming volume from the atria. At the end of diastole, the ventricles are at what is referred to as their "**end-diastolic volume**." The myocytes begin their contraction (systole) from this level of stretch. Since we cannot measure the length of an individual sarcomere, the volume of the ventricle provides us with a reasonable approximation of the stretch on the myocytes that make up the ventricle. Reflecting back on the original experiments that led to the length–tension concept, the ventricular end-diastolic volume is a three-dimensional representation of the individual sarcomere that was stretched prior to stimulation by an electrical impulse; greater stretch (represented by the volume of the ventricle) leads to a greater force of contraction.

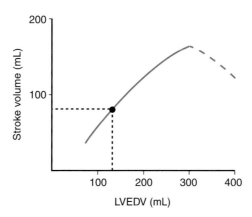

FIGURE 7-2 The ventricular function curve or Starling curve. This figure illustrates the important relationship between stroke volume (SV) and left ventricular end-diastolic volume (LVEDV). The intersecting dotted lines refer to the values of SV and EDV at rest. This illustrates the Frank–Starling relationship: under conditions of increased end-diastolic volume (increased ventricular filling), the heart muscle can develop greater tension and hence increased SV. The downward slope of the Starling curve at high EDV is controversial. Experimental studies show that this phenomenon can exist for isolated segments of the cardiac chamber; it is unclear whether the heart as a whole manifests a downward slope. Recall that the fibrous skeleton of the heart helps prevent overdistention of the muscle.

Thus, the left ventricular end-diastolic volume (LVEDV) determines, according to the length–tension relationship, the strength of the upcoming contraction.

This volume–contraction relationship is the basis of the Frank–Starling law of the heart. The design of the heart is very clever. *At rest*, the end-diastolic volume of the ventricle does not lead to the optimal level of overlap of myosin and actin (Panel B, *Figure* 7-1). In other words, the heart has reserve capacity; at rest, it is not operating at its maximal contractile capability. During exercise, for example, the volume of blood returning to the heart (called venous return) increases, and the LVEDV will be greater than normal. At an increased LVEDV, the ventricular wall will be subjected to increased stretch, will approach its optimal level of myofibril overlap, and, therefore, will generate more tension. Stroke volume, in response to the increased end-diastolic volume and increased force of contraction, will be enhanced. Simply stated, the Frank–Starling relationship indicates that "within reason, the heart will pump what it receives." *Figure* 7-2 illustrates this important relationship, called a **ventricular function curve** (or a Starling curve), between LVEDV (cardiac myocyte length) and SV (cardiac myocyte tension).

 Use Animated Figure 7-1 (Frank–Starling relationship) to explore the ventricular function curve. Vary the LVEDV to see the resultant changes in SV. You can also modify contractility (discussed extensively later in this chapter) and observe how such a change shifts the curve, thereby altering the relationship between LVEDV and SV. You may want to return to this figure as we discuss preload and contractility in the upcoming sections.

This intrinsic property of cardiac muscle is what ensures that any increased volume received by the right side of the heart is matched to a similar increased volume received by, and then pumped out from, the left ventricle. In other words, right heart output becomes the venous return to the left heart. Consequently, an increased venous return to the right ventricle leads to an increased SV and output from the right heart, which subsequently leads to increased venous return and output from the left ventricle. As we said above, under steady-state conditions, the output of the right and left ventricles must be matched.

Determinants of Cardiac Output

We have been discussing the relationship between end-diastolic volume and SV and have introduced the ventricular function curve. It is important now to elaborate further on three important cardiovascular concepts: preload, afterload, and contractility.

PRELOAD

Preload is the volume (load) filling the ventricle prior to contraction. For the left ventricle, the preload is represented by the LVEDV. When preload is increased, according to the Frank–Starling law, there will be a compensatory increase in SV. Various situations result in an increase in preload; for example, the addition of fluid to the circulation, either by transfusion of blood or by administration of salt solutions, is a very common clinical intervention to treat a patient who experiences a drop in blood pressure. One of the body's initial physiological responses to a drop in cardiac output is to constrict the veins, which reduces the reservoir capacity of the venous system and leads to a redistribution of blood from the venous to the arterial circulation. In both cases, administration of fluids and constriction of veins, there is an increase in venous return to the heart, which leads to increased preload. It is important to differentiate between preload and inotropy, both of which influence stroke volume. Changes in preload are associated with (and depend on) changes in end-diastolic volume. Changes in inotropy are independent of the level of end-diastolic volume and are associated with changes in SNS activity (more on this later in the chapter).

Another way to visualize preload and its effects on stroke volume is through the use of the pressure volume loop (*Figure 7-3*). To review, at point A (end-systolic volume), the mitral valve opens and blood returns to the relaxed left ventricle. At point B, the ventricle begins to contract, pressure rises, and the mitral valve closes (beginning isovolumetric contraction). At point C, the aortic valve opens and ventricular ejection begins; left ventricular volume now falls. At point D, the aortic valve closes and the ventricle relaxes (isovolumetric relaxation). Stroke volume, therefore, is the difference, on the *X*-axis, between points C (end-diastolic volume) and D (end-systolic volume). Preload, using this diagram,

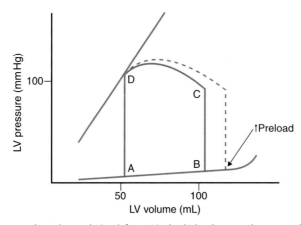

FIGURE 7-3 This is a pressure volume loop relating left ventricular (LV) volume and pressure through one cycle of systole and diastole. The solid line represents the normal condition, and the dashed line illustrates the changes to this loop with an increase in preload. The greater LVEDV elicits a stronger contraction (Frank–Starling law) and greater stroke volume (C to D).

is represented by the ventricular volume at point B, or the amount of filling (mL) prior to isovolumetric contraction. As mentioned in our discussion of the Frank–Starling law, an increase in preload (represented by the shift of point B to the right) will increase stroke volume (C would also be shifted to the right).

 Animated Figure 7-2 (PV loop and preload) illustrates preload in the context of the pressure volume loop. Change the preload (here represented by the LVEDV on the horizontal axis) and note the corresponding change in the PV loop. An isolated increase in preload leads to an increase in SV, whereas a decrease in preload decreases SV; in both cases, the end-systolic volume (labeled as ESV) does not change.

> **THOUGHT QUESTION 7-1:** You are sitting in a room for 10 minutes; you decide to meditate to slow your heart. Your heart rate goes from 80 to 60 beats/min; assuming CO stays the same, what would happen to preload and why?

AFTERLOAD

Afterload is an important but slightly less intuitive concept. After the left ventricle is filled with blood (end diastole), it contracts, and, when LV pressure exceeds the pressure downstream of the aortic valve, ejects blood into the aorta (review Chapter 4 on the cardiac cycle if you need a refresher on valve function). We refer to the stress in the ventricular wall necessary to generate the pressure required to open the aortic valve and eject its stroke volume as the afterload. You may also hear the term "ventricular wall tension" used synonymously with **ventricular wall stress**. Wall stress is a measure of the load that is distributed over the muscle fibers in the ventricular wall. Higher wall stress than normal indicates that each muscle fiber bears a greater load; conversely, lower wall stress indicates that each muscle fiber bears a lesser overall load. According to Laplace's law, wall stress is equal to the product of the ventricular transmural (across the wall) pressure (P) times the radius of the chamber (r), divided by 2 times the wall thickness (h).

$$\text{Wall stress} = (P \cdot r)/2\,h$$

The easiest way to begin to understand wall stress is to change one variable at a time in Laplace's law. If the radius and wall thickness are held constant, then wall stress varies directly with the intraventricular pressure needed to open the aortic valve (note: the intraventricular pressure equals the transmural pressure when the pressure outside the ventricle is 0, i.e., equal to atmospheric pressure; the pressure outside the ventricle is approximately equal to the pericardial pressure, which is near zero in the absence of cardiopulmonary disease). If pressure is held constant, on the other hand, and the radius of the ventricle increases, greater wall stress will be necessary to generate the same pressure.

 Use Animated Figure 7-3 (Laplace's law and wall stress) to alter each variable in Laplace's law, shown for the left ventricular wall, and observe the changes in wall stress. Notice that elevated pressure is associated with higher wall stress, that is, each muscle fiber must exert more force to generate the higher pressure if chamber radius and wall thickness are unchanged. Increasing wall thickness (accomplished by hypertrophy of the muscle), with other variables held constant, decreases wall stress because the load is distributed across a greater number of muscle sarcomeres.

EDITOR'S INTEGRATION
We use the concept of "transmural pressure" when defining afterload because of
the effect of pleural or pericardial pressure on the heart in certain disease states.
The transmural pressure of a flexible three-dimensional object is the pressure
inside the object minus the pressure outside the object. If the heart is being
squeezed by a high pressure surrounding the ventricle (either because of increased
pressure in the pleural space or the pericardium), then the pressure generated
inside the ventricle reflects a combination of forces generated by contraction of
the myocytes and by the pericardium or chest wall. In cardiac tamponade,
for example, a condition characterized by the accumulation of fluid in the
pericardium, an intraventricular pressure of 120 mm Hg may be the consequence
of pressure created by the fluid and by ventricular contraction; thus, wall stress
would be less than if the pressure were created solely by contraction of the
myocytes. The concept of transmural pressure is critical for determining preload
of the ventricles in patients with respiratory failure treated with mechanical
ventilators and for understanding the factors that determine lung volume
(see Chapter 3, "Respiratory Physiology: A Clinical Approach").

The pressure in the aorta (or the arterial blood pressure) is a close approximation of the afterload, but it should not be viewed as equivalent to afterload. To do so will result in mistakes when you consider what happens to patients with heart disease, impaired cardiac output, and those treated with drugs that dilate arteries. We will illustrate this point by discussing treatment of a patient who has heart failure, a dilated ventricle, and a low cardiac output. Cardiac output is governed by the following equation (analogoue to Ohm's Law that you learned in physics and discussed further in chapter 9)

$$MAP - CVP = CO \times SVR$$

(where MAP = Mean arterial pressure, CVP = Central venous pressure, CO = Cardiac output, and SVR is systemic vascular resistance). You decide to initiate therapy with a drug that reduces SVR and often leads to a fall in blood pressure (typically called a vasodilator or "afterload reducer") in an effort to increase cardiac output. If cardiac output goes up proportionately to the fall in SVR, however, blood pressure (MAP) will stay the same. If you equated afterload with blood pressure, you would conclude that you had not reduced the afterload with this medication and that it was mislabeled. In reality, however, the medication did reduce afterload by enhancing stroke volume. The increase in stroke volume reduced the radius of the ventricle, thereby diminishing wall stress per Laplace's Law.

A person with chronically high arterial pressure has an elevated afterload. In other words, the heart must generate higher left ventricular pressure (and therefore wall stress) in order to exceed the aortic pressure, open the aortic valve, and eject the stroke volume. When an individual has high blood pressure for months to years, the heart responds by thickening the muscle wall, a process called **hypertrophy**. The wall thickening (or the increase in "*h*" in the Laplace equation) is a compensatory mechanism to reduce wall stress. The type of thickening you see with increased pressure load is called **concentric hypertrophy**. Cardiac hypertrophy in hypertension is the consequence of a process similar to the enlargement of your biceps muscle when you have been following an exercise routine that includes training with heavy weights; the body responds to the stress associated with generating increased pressure by adding contractile fibers to the muscle. In contrast, a dilated ventricle with increased radius also has increased wall stress (e.g., as seen in patients with mitral regurgitation who must pump more blood on each beat because part of the stroke volume goes backwards into the atrium); however, this leads to a different type of hypertrophy called eccentric hypertrophy, which involves less thickening and more

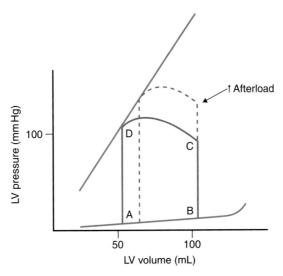

FIGURE 7-4 This is a pressure volume loop relating left ventricular (LV) volume and pressure through one cycle of systole and diastole. The solid line represents the normal condition, and the dashed line illustrates the changes to this loop with an increase in afterload. As afterload increases, the heart must spend more time during systole in isometric contraction; less time is available for ejection and stroke volume (C, D) is reduced.

chamber dilation. The condition of chronic high arterial pressure represents "pressure work" (high pressure, normal or low stroke volume) for the ventricle; the condition of mitral regurgitation represents "volume work" (high stroke volume with normal or low pressure). Although both represent problems that increase wall stress, the body compensates in different ways to minimize afterload and the oxygen needs of the myocardium.

The concept of afterload can be illustrated using the pressure volume loop (*Figure* 7-4). Afterload can be approximated as the pressure achieved at point C, when the aortic valve opens. In the context of an abrupt increase in afterload (e.g., increased arterial pressure due to vasoconstriction), an increased left ventricular pressure (LVP) would be required to open the aortic valve and, thus, would result in an increase in the height of the line between points B and C. To overcome the increased pressure required to open the aortic valve, the myocytes must spend more time in isometric contraction, which leaves less time and energy for cardiac muscle fiber shortening; consequently, less blood is ejected from the left ventricle. On the pressure volume curve, this series of events would translate into reaching point D at a higher left ventricular volume (i.e., decreased stroke volume).

 Animated Figure 7-4 (PV loop and afterload) uses the pressure volume loop to illustrate the concept of afterload. Change the afterload (here represented by the C point on the PV loop) and note the corresponding change in the PV loop. An isolated increase in afterload leads to a decreased SV, whereas a decrease in afterload increases SV. This diagram represents the effects on the cardiac cycle immediately after an abrupt change in afterload. How the heart compensates in the short term (the subsequent cardiac cycles) is discussed in detail shortly.

We can characterize the changes outlined above with the concept of **ejection fraction** (the percentage of blood ejected with each heart beat).

$$EF = SV/EDV$$

where EF is ejection fraction, SV is stroke volume, and EDV is end-diastolic volume. We observed that increased afterload reduces stroke volume. We can now relate that to ejection fraction. Afterload is inversely related to the velocity of myocardial fiber shortening; if afterload is increased, the amount of fiber shortening is diminished, and the consequence is a reduction in ejection fraction. Stated in another way, if one considers the time allotted for contraction of the myocyte, part of systole is devoted to isovolumetric contraction (generating pressure to open the aortic valve) and part to isotonic contraction (ejecting the blood into the aorta). As aortic pressure increases, a greater fraction of systole must be devoted to isovolumetric contraction. This results in a reduction in SV and ejection fraction; consequently, there is more blood left in the ventricle after systole, leading to an increase in end-systolic volume.

During the next diastole, blood returns to the left ventricle and is added to the increased left ventricular end-systolic volume (LVESV), resulting in a higher than normal end-diastolic volume. As long as the heart is healthy, this increased end-diastolic volume (EDV) will (via the Frank–Starling law) result in an increased SV compared to the previous contraction; thus SV has been restored to near normal, although the end-systolic volume is now elevated. If this is occurring in a heart with compromised pumping ability, however, the heart may have to dilate significantly more to try to achieve the normal stroke volume; this may come at the expense of a major increase in afterload associated with a very large ventricular radius. The ejection fraction will be reduced under these circumstances (stroke volume may be near normal, but EDV is increased). This new steady state of over filling and increased wall stress persists for some time but eventually can lead to heart failure (see below).

Animated Figure 7-5 (PV loop and afterload—acute progression) shows the changes in the PV loop over the cardiac cycles immediately following an abrupt increase in afterload. Play the sequence and notice how the SV is initially reduced by the increased afterload, but is partially restored by the subsequent increase in preload. The result is a ventricle operating at higher pressures and volumes than normal, both of which contribute to increased wall stress.

It is important to remember that chronic exposure to high afterload makes the ventricle work harder than normal. As we discussed above, the heart, like any muscle that is exposed to a greater workload, will increase its mass, that is, hypertrophy, over time. At first blush this may sound like a good (and adaptive) response, and initially it is. The increased ventricular wall thickness reduces the ventricular wall stress (or afterload) and helps maintain the cardiac output.

$$\downarrow wall\ stress = (P \cdot r)\ /\uparrow h$$

Unfortunately, the cellular nature of the hypertrophic changes in ventricular muscle can interfere with calcium handling (among other things); over time, if the hypertrophy goes unchecked, the ventricle becomes a less and less efficient pump. Eventually, these changes may lead to heart failure.

Animated Figure 7-6 (Concentric hypertrophy and wall stress) illustrates the hypertrophy that results from an extended period of elevated afterload. Use the diagram to watch each stage of the progression; the first stage shown combines Animated Figures 7-4 and 7-5. Watch the hypertrophy stage to see how increased thickness of the ventricular wall leads to decreased wall stress. Despite this, concentric hypertrophy is not a state that can be maintained indefinitely without consequences; the final stage of the figure shows the progression to heart failure that may occur if the condition causing the elevated afterload (e.g., hypertension or aortic stenosis) is left untreated.

A heart in "failure" has a much flatter ventricular function curve (*Figure* 7-5 and Animated Figure 7-1); the curve is shifted downward, which means that for any given LVEDV, the stroke volume and cardiac output are reduced when compared to the normal state. As described above, the increased volume of blood that remains in the ventricles and atria following contractions of an impaired ventricle leads to increased end-diastolic filling and pressure (point i to point ii in *Figure* 7-5). This is a physiological response to try to preserve stroke volume and cardiac output, but in heart failure the result is an insignificant rise in SV. In addition, the increase in EDV results in adverse cardiorespiratory consequences. To get blood to flow from the left atrium to left ventricle, left atrial pressure must increase; to get

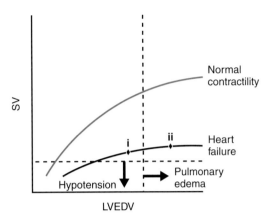

FIGURE 7-5 Ventricular function curve in heart failure. This illustrates the relationship between left ventricular end-diastolic volume (LVEDV) and stroke volume (SV) in a normal individual and a person with systolic heart failure. Notice how flat the curve is in the person with heart failure; increasing end-diastolic volume in these patients does little to increase stroke volume.

blood flow from the pulmonary veins to the left atrium, pulmonary venous pressure must increase. The final result is increased hydrostatic pressure in the pulmonary capillaries and movement of fluid across the capillaries and into the interstitium of the lung as well as the alveoli; in some cases, this may lead to a serious medical condition called pulmonary edema.

Not all forms of hypertrophy, however, result in the deleterious effects described above. We have all heard about elite level athletes, training for 5 hours a day, who have hypertrophied hearts. According to Frey and Olson (2003) athletic (physiological) and pathological hypertrophy differ both morphologically and at the molecular level. Some changes seen in pathological (but not physiological) hypertrophy include

- Diastolic filling is impaired (because of increased fibrosis).
- Capillarity is decreased (muscle mass increases but the number of blood vessels in the muscle stays the same, which results in decreased density of capillaries per gram of muscle).
- There is a shift toward an apoptotic (programmed cell death) pathway.
- The increased cardiac mass leads to arrhythmias.
- There is an increased susceptibility to injury after ischemia or reperfusion.

In addition, physiological hypertrophy typically is not accompanied by an accumulation of myocardial collagen, does not exceed a modest level of ventricular wall thickness, and is not accompanied by different expression of several "hypertrophic genes" (as is seen in pathological hypertrophy).

CONTRACTILITY

We think of **contractility** as a change in the heart's strength of contraction for any given level of end-diastolic volume (or preload). If you look at the ventricular function curve (*Figure 7-6*), you will see that an increase in contractility shifts the curve up and to the left over the entire range of end-diastolic volumes. In contrast, a decrease in contractility shifts the normal curve down and to the right such that you have less SV across the range of end-diastolic volume.

Both norepinephrine and epinephrine increase cardiac contractility; this is a key component of the "fight or flight response," which requires the body to quickly increase cardiac output. Drugs that alter contractility either up or down are called "inotropic" agents. A drug that increases contractility (e.g., digoxin, dobutamine) is called a positive inotrope,

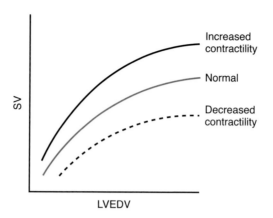

FIGURE 7-6 Ventricular function curve. Increasing contractility shifts the normal ventricular function curve up and to the left such that you have greater stroke volume (SV) across the range of left ventricular end-diastolic volume (EDV). In contrast, a decrease in contractility shifts the normal curve down and to the right such that you have less SV across the range of EDV.

whereas a drug that depresses contractility (e.g., calcium channel blockers) is called a negative inotrope. The consequence of an increase in contractility (positive inotropy) is a greater SV and ejection fraction (which implies a decreased end-systolic volume compared to the conditions prior to the change in contractility). As with the fight or flight response, this is particularly important during exercise when the increased level of sympathetic stimulation increases contractility. In exercise, contraction of the active muscles compresses the veins and leads to increased venous return, which increases end-diastolic volume; because of the associated increase in contractility, however, stroke volume increases in absolute terms and end-systolic volume may be normal or lower than normal. In addition, enhanced lusitropy permits increased diastolic filling during exercise. Without the combined positive inotropic and lusitropic effects associated with increased sympathetic stimulation, the exercise-induced elevation in HR, which reduces the duration of diastole, could decrease diastolic filling and SV.

> **? THOUGHT QUESTION 7-2: A patient arrives at the ED complaining of shortness of breath at rest and with exertion. He is having trouble breathing when he lies down, and he is waking up at night with labored breathing. He is diagnosed with heart failure and given a positive inotrope (digoxin or dobutamine). Describe the physiological changes associated with this therapy that will benefit this patient?**

Changes in contractility can also be demonstrated using the pressure volume loop (*Figure* 7-7). In this scenario, if we keep aortic pressure and preload constant but increase contractility, you start at the same point C (opening of the aortic valve) but because there is an increased strength of contraction you empty the ventricle more fully, leaving a lower end-systolic volume (shifting point D to a lower LV end-systolic volume). The result is a larger stroke volume (distance from C to D).

Use Animated Figure 7-7 (PV loop and contractility) to vary contractility. As mentioned above, if we hold preload and aortic valve opening pressure (our surrogate for afterload) constant, an increase in contractility increases stroke volume and ejection fraction. Conversely, if you decrease contractility in the figure (again with preload and afterload held constant), you can see how the rightward and downward shift of the end-systolic pressure volume relationship (ESPVR) leads to a decrease in SV and EF.

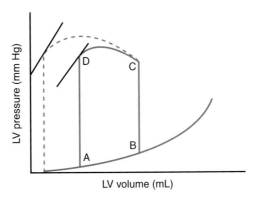

FIGURE 7-7 This is a pressure volume loop relating left ventricular (LV) volume and pressure through one cycle of systole and diastole. The solid line represents the normal condition, and the dashed line illustrates the changes to this loop with an increase in contractility (while holding preload constant). Stroke volume (C to D) is increased, which results in a smaller end-systolic volume.

Measurement

CARDIAC OUTPUT

To measure cardiac output you can use one of two techniques. One method is called the **indicator dilution method**. This utilizes a special flow-directed pulmonary artery catheter called a "Swan–Ganz" catheter, so named after its inventors Jeremy Swan and William Ganz (these catheters are generically known now as "pulmonary artery catheters"). The Swan–Ganz catheter has a balloon at its forward tip; when inflated with air, the balloon tip of the catheter is carried by the venous blood flow through the right atrium and ventricle and ultimately into the pulmonary artery. Apparently, Jeremy Swan got the idea for a flow-directed catheter while watching the wind playing with the sails on a sailboat and he imagined a catheter "sailing through the heart."

The indicator dilution method for estimating cardiac output is based on the assumption that the flow (mL/min) of blood can be calculated when a measurable indicator substance is delivered upstream of the right ventricle, mixes with the blood in the RV, and is remeasured (after dilution with blood) in the pulmonary artery. The substance often used is "cooled saline," and it can be delivered and measured (by assessing the temperature of the blood) using the pulmonary artery catheter. This technique, when using a thermal indicator, is called thermodilution.

Animated Figure 7-8 (Thermodilution for measuring cardiac output) illustrates the basic idea of how cooled saline can be used to determine cardiac output.

The second method of estimating cardiac output makes use of a principle discovered by Adolf Eugene Fick (and named after him as "the Fick principle"). The concept is based on the observation that the total uptake or release of a substance by a given organ is the product of the blood flow of the organ multiplied by the difference in the content of the substance in the arterial and venous blood going to and returning from that organ. When the substance being measured is oxygen, the uptake is known as $\dot{V}O_2$ (mL/min). To assess the cardiac output using the Fick principle, we measure the oxygen consumption by determining how much oxygen a person breathes in and out (the difference is the amount consumed by the tissue). The arterial content of the blood (CaO2) is determined by obtaining a sample from an artery, typically the radial artery. The content of oxygen in the venous blood (CvO2) must be taken from a place that mixes blood returning from all regions of the body; the blood in the pulmonary artery, which can be accessed from the tip of the Swan–Ganz catheter, provides a "mixed venous" sample. With these data in hand, we can calculate the cardiac output (CO) as follows:

$$\text{Oxygen delivered to the tissue} - \text{Oxygen returned from tissue} = \text{Oxygen consumed } \dot{V}O_2$$

$$CO \times CaO2 - CO \times CvO2 = \dot{V}O2$$

$$CO\ (CaO2 - CvO2) = \dot{V}O2$$

$$CO\ (\text{L/min}) = \frac{\dot{V}O_2\ (\text{mLO}_2/\text{min})}{[CaO2 - CvO2]\ (\text{mLO}_2/\text{L})}$$

EJECTION FRACTION

As we described earlier, another important cardiovascular measurement that provides information about cardiac function is the **ejection fraction**. This is the percentage of the blood in the ventricle at the end of diastole (end-diastolic volume) that is ejected (ejected blood is the stroke volume).

$$\text{Ejection fraction (EF)} = \frac{\text{End-diastolic volume} - \text{End-systolic volume}}{\text{End-diastolic volume}}$$

Since Stroke volume = End-diastolic volume − End-systolic volume,

$$EF = \frac{\text{Stroke volume}}{\text{End-diastolic volume}}$$

Normal range of EF is 55% to 70%. People with systolic heart failure can have EF values of well below 55%, while EF is much higher during exercise; patients with diastolic dysfunction (impaired relaxation of the ventricle) may exhibit symptoms of heart failure with normal EF. Ejection fraction can be measured noninvasively; two methods, **echocardiography** and **radionucleotide ventriculography** (RVG), are commonly used clinically. Echocardiography utilizes sound waves to produce a moving image of the heart and its chambers and valves. Radio nucleotide ventriculography utilizes radioactively-labeled red blood cells and a gamma camera to image the heart and provide a direct volumetric assessment of the cardiac chambers throughout the cardiac cycle; this test is known for its high reproducibility and low interobserver and intraobserver variability.

PUTTING IT TOGETHER

It is the middle of the night and you are a volunteer in the emergency department (ED) when Margaret Leung (32 years old) is brought in by ambulance from her home. Over the last few months she has become progressively more and more fatigued and tonight she woke up in a panic, feeling as if she couldn't breathe (this sudden shortness of breath at night is called "paroxysmal nocturnal dyspnea"). She says she has had a persistent cough, which gets worse (as does her breathing) a couple of hours after she lies down to sleep at night (shortness of breath that worsens in the supine position is called "orthopnea"). Her blood pressure is low, and her HR is high. The ED doctor listens to her chest and says she hears evidence of fluid in her lungs. When lungs are filled with interstitial fluid, they become stiffer or less compliant and there is a predisposition to collapse of small airways and alveoli; during inspiration, these collapsed structures reexpand and the sudden equalization of pressures that occurs between the collapsed and open central airways as they "pop" open produce a crackling sound called "moist rales."

Review Questions

1. A patient is treated with a drug that mimics the effect of adrenergic stimulation (e.g., a β-receptor agonist) and, as a result, the stroke volume has changed. The result could best be described by which of the following terms?
    A. Negative chronotropic effect
    B. Negative inotropic effect
    C. Positive inotropic and lusitropic effects
    D. Negative inotropic and lusitropic effects

2. A patient under your care has suffered a myocardial infarction, with some residual heart muscle damage, and has a diminished ejection fraction. While still in the hospital his blood pressure falls to 80/40 mm Hg, his HR drops to 35 beats/min, and an ECG shows he is in third degree heart block (no electrical connection between his atria and ventricles); he has low urine output, and his jugular venous pulse is normal. A resident, reacting to the low blood pressure and urine output, suggests an IV administration of saline to bolster his blood pressure.
    What would you predict would be the outcome of giving the IV saline to this patient?
    A. Decreasing afterload and increasing cardiac output
    B. Decreasing preload and further hypotension
    C. Increasing preload and pulmonary edema
    D. Increasing systemic vascular resistance and afterload

3. A 65-year-old man suffers from recurrent fainting episodes (syncope). In your review of his medical history, you discovered that he has moderate dementia and stable asthma. He is taking galantamine (an acetylcholinesterase inhibitor) and a multivitamin regularly, and he uses inhalers occasionally. His physical examination was normal except for heart rate of 45 beats/min. You believe his recurrent syncope is due to symptomatic bradycardia resulting from his galantamine. What is the best explanation of the mechanism by which this drug would have this effect?
    A. Decrease parasympathetic nervous system (PSNS) effect on heart rate due to decreased acetylcholine level in the SA node.
    B. Decrease sympathetic nervous system (SNS) effect on heart rate due to decreased acetylcholine level in the SA node
    C. Increase PSNS effect on heart rate due to increased acetylcholine level in the SA node
    D. Increase SNS effect on heart rate due to increased acetylcholine level in the SA node

4. In heart failure, for a given left ventricular end-diastolic volume (LVEDV), the stroke volume (SV) on the Starling curve, compared to normal conditions, will be:
    A. Higher
    B. Lower

5. A 75-year-old man was being treated for heart failure and pulmonary edema. Which of the following treatments would not be beneficial for this patient?
    A. Calcium channel blocker
    B. Dobutamine
    C. Oxygen supplementation
    D. IV loop diuretics

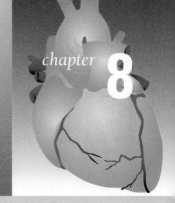

chapter 8

Blood Vessels:
Special Delivery

CHAPTER OUTLINE

LEARNING OBJECTIVES

By the end of the chapter you will be able to:
- Relate the structure and function of the major classifications of blood vessels in the circulatory system (arteries, veins, capillaries, and lymph).
- Describe the Starling forces and how they apply to the development of both pulmonary and systemic edema.
- Describe the role for excitation–contraction (EC) coupling in vascular smooth muscle and its relationship to changes in vascular resistance.
- Describe and give examples of the following factors that affect arteriolar diameter: neural, humoral, endothelial, tissue metabolites, and myogenic factors.
- Explain the underlying mechanism of autoregulation.
- Differentiate between the distinguishing features of and regulatory mechanisms that operate on the following circulations: cerebral circulation, coronary circulation, and pulmonary circulation.
- Define angiogenesis and explain the mechanisms that promotes or inhibits it.

Introduction

It's all very well for the heart to be the powerhouse of the circulatory system pumping blood to the body, but we need a system to deliver blood, which carries oxygen and nutrients to and removes waste from the tissues of the body; we must have an intricate network of tubes or vessels to link the pump to the metabolically active cells. Vessels are incredibly designed to fulfill different functions; some are made for fast delivery, some constrict and dilate and function as gatekeepers for blood delivery, and some are thin walled and promote exchange of gases and nutrients. There is even a system of vessels that is named after the fluid they carry, lymph, which is leaked into the interstitial space. The role of the lymph vessels is to return this fluid to the vasculature.

Smooth muscle in the walls of vessels contributes to the control of blood pressure and to the change in vessel diameter that occurs in response to a variety of neural and hormonal factors. Certain organs, including the brain, heart, and lungs, have special features within their vascular beds that ensure they are always adequately perfused; the processes that enable the vessels to alter their size and resistance to flow in response to external factors are called "autoregulation." Under special circumstances, the body can even grow additional blood vessels, a process called "angiogenesis," to ensure that the supply of blood and nutrients is matched to demand.

Characterizing the Body's Vessels

Blood vessels are designed to link structure and function. You can classify vessels into the following categories:

- conduit vessels that transport blood quickly to and from regions of the body (e.g., aorta, vena cavae);
- distribution vessels that distribute and return blood specifically to and from various organs. Distribution vessels tend to have names (e.g., femoral artery or brachial vein) that relate to the organ or structure they serve;
- resistance vessels (e.g., arterioles) that account for the bulk of the resistance in the circulation;
- exchange vessels (e.g., capillaries) that allow for the movement of gases, fluids, and nutrients into and out of the blood;
- capacitance vessels (e.g., veins) that act as a reservoir for blood. These vessels can hold a large amount of volume at a low pressure, a characteristic of structures with high compliance (recall $C = \Delta V/\Delta P$);
- and finally lymph vessels that help maintain fluid balance. These vessels absorb the fluid and small proteins lost in the interstitial spaces and return them to the vascular system.

All vessels have a basic architecture with three layers (or a subset of these three layers): intima, media, and adventitia (see *Figure* 8-1).

The **tunica intima** is the layer that is in contact with (or most intimate with) the blood. It consists of a continuous layer of endothelial cells that connect end-to-end to form the lumen of the blood vessel. The "tightness" of the connections between endothelial cells can determine the leakiness of the vessel and its capacity for the exchange of small molecules (e.g., cerebral vessels have virtually no exchange across the so-called "blood–brain barrier"; in contrast, the liver or kidney vessels have large pores with capacity for significant exchange). It is within the intima of vessels that **endothelin** (a vasoconstrictor) and **nitric oxide** (NO) (a vasodilator) are synthesized and released. The balance between the actions of these hormones on the vascular smooth muscle in the tunica media contributes to changes in resistance and, hence, flow of blood through the vessel.

The **tunica media** contains vascular smooth muscle, the cells of which are connected to each other, end-to-end, circumferentially around the vessel. When they contract, they pull in on the vessel. This process, termed "**vasoconstriction**," plays an important role in

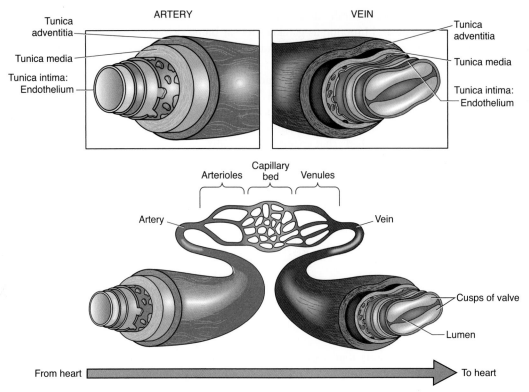

FIGURE 8-1 The structure of blood vessels. This figure illustrates the three basic layers (or tunics) of most blood vessels. The innermost layer, the tunica intima, consists primarily of endothelial cells and a basement membrane. The middle layer, the tunica media, comprises smooth muscle cells and elastic tissue, and the outermost layer, the tunica adventitia, is a fibrous tissue covering. With the exception of capillaries (which do not contain smooth muscle), blood vessels have all three layers.

regulation of vascular resistance and, hence, blood pressure. As you will see, constriction of veins (**venoconstriction**) is also an important regulator of venous return, the flow of blood back to the heart. Conversely, **vasodilation** or **venodilation** relaxes the vascular smooth muscle and allows increased blood to flow through the arteries and a pooling of blood in the veins. The media also contains elastic tissue, which contributes to something called "elastic recoil" (see the following text).

The **tunica adventitia (or tunica externa)** is the outer layer of the blood vessel and consists of connective tissue, small arteries, and autonomic nerves. You might think that blood vessel walls would get their blood supply from the blood running within their lumen. Although that might be true of the very smallest vessels, most of the large, thick-walled vessels contain tiny blood vessels that penetrate into their muscular walls; these are called "**vaso vasorum**." The vaso vasorum supply oxygen and nourishment to the thick muscular walls of the vessels. In addition, autonomic nerves permeate the media to act directly on the vascular smooth muscle, thereby regulating vasodilation and vasoconstriction.

Now that you know what makes up the blood vessels, we can distinguish among the vessels functionally by observing the proportion of each of the three layers within the wall of any given type of vessel.

Let's start with conduit/transportation vessels, using the aorta as an example. The wall of the aorta contains all three layers. It is a large blood vessel with two major functions, (a) to move blood at high pressure, away from the heart and (b) using something called "**elastic** recoil," to bolster blood pressure between contractions of the left ventricle i.e., during diastole. The structural features that help it to carry out its two functions include a large diameter (30 mm), which reduces resistance and contributes to fast delivery of blood, and thick muscular walls with elastic tissue in the media. This second feature is the key to sustaining diastolic blood pressure. During systole, the elastic fibers in the walls allow the aorta to expand to accept the powerful expulsion of blood from the ventricle. As systole ends and the ventricle relaxes, the expanded walls recoil, thereby maintaining blood pressure during the diastolic period between contractions of the heart.

> **?**
>
> **THOUGHT QUESTION 8-1:** How would the flow of blood through the arteries be changed if the arteries were rigid pipes rather than elastic structures, and how does this explain why elderly patients have a widened pulse pressure (pulse pressure = systolic pressure [SP] – diastolic pressure [DP])?

Distribution arteries have all three layers but fewer elastic fibers in the walls than are found in the aorta. They have a liberal amount of vascular smooth muscle within their media, which allows them to constrict and dilate to alter distribution of cardiac output to various vascular beds.

Under normal physiological conditions; however, it is the arterioles or resistance vessels that are primarily responsible for changes in blood flow to different organs. They respond to the various needs of the body under different circumstances. For example, during exercise, when you want blood to go primarily to the exercising muscles and not to the kidney or gut, the arterioles within the muscles dilate while those serving the gut and kidney constrict. These actions insure that proportionally more of the cardiac output will go to the exercising muscles to meet their metabolic needs. The resistance vessels are very small vessels whose main function is to constrict or dilate in order to manipulate the resistance to blood flow and, hence, the systemic blood pressure. They have a relatively large amount of vascular smooth muscle for their size. In a situation in which blood pressure falls acutely (a bleeding ulcer as one example), the sympathetic nervous system is stimulated, which leads to vasoconstriction at the level of the systemic arterioles. The resultant increase in resistance (systemic vascular resistance) helps to bolster the fallen blood pressure since:

$$MAP - CVP = CO \times SVR$$

(MAP, mean arterial pressure; CVP, central venous pressure; CO, cardiac output; SVR, systemic vascular resistance; more detail in Chapter 9).

Vasoconstriction during an activity such as exercise, which is associated with increased sympathetic nervous system activity, does not result in an increase in systemic vascular resistance, as occurs in the case of a bleeding ulcer, because of the additional effects of local mediators of vascular tone in exercising muscles. During exercise, blood vessels to the abdomen (kidney and gut) constrict, whereas blood vessels to the exercising muscles dilate; the latter is a consequence of local hypoxia and the accumulation of metabolic products in the tissue (more detail on this later in chapter). The net effect is that systemic vascular resistance actually falls. Blood pressure during exercise is maintained due to the increase in heart rate (HR) and stroke volume (SV), which results in a rise in CO, thereby compensating for the fall in SVR.

Exchange vessels, or capillaries (*Figure 8-2*), are unique among vessels in the body in that they consist solely of a layer of endothelial cells linked end-to-end to form a tube. The

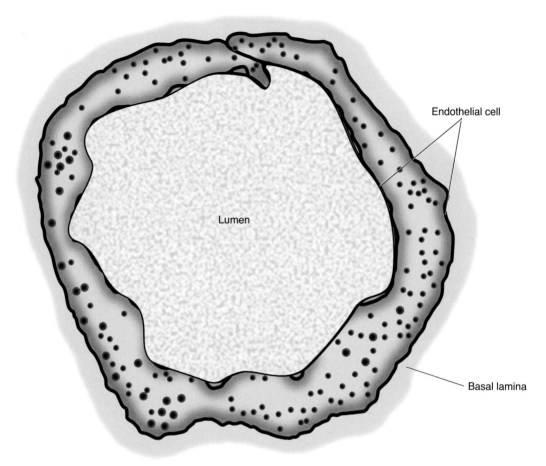

Endothelial cell

Lumen

Basal lamina

FIGURE 8-2 Capillary in cross section. This figure of a histological image shows a capillary in cross section; note the thin wall made up of endothelial cells and surrounded by a basal lamina. The structures inside the endothelial cell are membrane-bound cytoplasmic vesicles.

endothelial cells and associated pericytes (mesenchymal cells that produce cytokines and growth factors not shown in Figure 8-2) are surrounded by a basal lamina (no media, no adventitia). An important function of the endothelial cells is to allow exchange of oxygen, carbon dioxide, nutrients, fluid, and small proteins; they also produce nitric oxide and endothelin, which are important factors in the regulation of vascular tone. Normal capillaries fall into three categories, which are determined by the tightness of the junctions between the endothelial cells. **Continuous capillaries** (e.g., those found in the brain, lung, muscle) allow little to no exchange across the tight junctions that form between the endothelial cells. The basement membrane is intact in these capillaries. **Fenestrated capillaries** (e.g., those found in kidneys, intestinal villi, endocrine glands) have small pores (fenestrae) between endothelial cells and allow the passage of small substances across the membrane. Lastly, the **discontinuous capillaries**, which are also known as sinusoids, have many large gaps between the endothelial cells and within the basement membrane. These are the leakiest capillaries; they are found in the liver, spleen, and bone marrow.

Veins, like arteries, contain all three structural layers (intima, media, and adventitia) but have relatively thin walls compared to arteries. There is proportionally less smooth muscle in the media of the veins, which gives them a floppy (as opposed to rigid) consistency. We call them "capacitance vessels," which means they have the "capacity" to hold a large volume of blood at a relatively low pressure. In other words, they have a high compliance and are capable of expanding their diameter to accommodate increased volume without a significant rise in pressure. In fact, under normal conditions at rest, 70% of the body's blood is contained in the veins. This comes in handy in situations in which there is a need to bolster the blood pressure by shifting volume from the veins into the arterial system. The veins constrict (as a result of sympathetic nerve activity), which forces blood back to the heart and into the systemic circulation. It's like getting a transfusion of blood from within our own body. It is also important to understand that, unlike large arteries with pulsatile pressure changes (as a result of contraction of the ventricles), large veins have a constant lower pressure throughout the cardiac cycle. The presence of unidirectional valves helps to promote forward flow toward the heart (particularly in the leg veins that need to overcome gravity to return blood to the heart). Breakdown of the walls of veins or valve dysfunction results in a condition, called "varicose veins," in which the surface veins become distended and tortuous. This condition is often painful and debilitating.

In addition to having valves, veins also utilize something called the "**skeletal muscle pump**" to facilitate blood flow at low pressure back to the heart against gravity (*Figure 8-3*). Veins (particularly in the legs) are surrounded by skeletal muscle which, when contracted, squeezes the veins. Since the valves prevent backward flow, the blood is propelled forward to the heart. This is the rationale for the advice to flex your leg muscles if you have to stand in a stationary position for any length of time; soldiers standing at attention for prolonged periods have been known to lose consciousness because of the pooling of blood in the leg veins and consequent drop in blood pressure. Remember this when you are standing still and assisting during a lengthy procedure in the operating room!

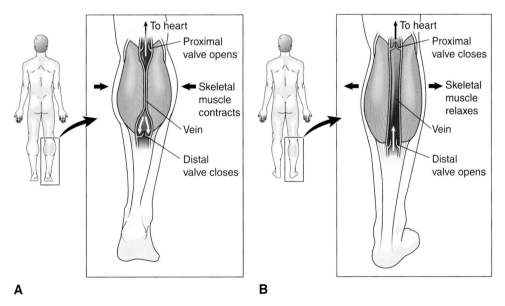

A   **B**

FIGURE 8-3 The skeletal muscle pump. The enlarged image of the lower leg shows a vein containing one-way valves, surrounded by a band of skeletal muscle; when the muscle contracts, it squeezes the vein and propels the blood toward the heart. When the skeletal muscle is relaxed, blood once again fills the vein. From Cohen BJ, Taylor JJ. *Memmler's The Human Body in Health and Disease.* 10th ed. Baltimore, MD: Lippincott Williams & Wilkins; 2005.

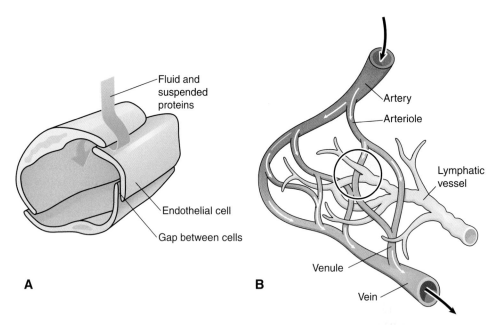

FIGURE 8-4 The lymphatics. This figure shows a single lymphatic vessel (panel **A**) with its overlapping and loosely connected endothelial walls; this construction allows interstitial fluid to move into the lymphatic vessel where it contributes to lymph fluid. Panel **B** shows a network of arterioles (in red), venules (in gray), and lymph vessels (in pink) and their relationship to the surrounding interstitial cells. Lymphatic vessels start as blind-ended tubes and join together to form larger and larger lymphatic vessels. From Cohen BJ, Taylor JJ. *Memmler's The Human Body in Health and Disease.* 10th ed. Baltimore, MD: Lippincott Williams & Wilkins; 2005.

The last category of vessels is the lymph vessels (*Figure* 8-4). These vessels share structural similarity to both veins and capillaries. Like veins, they are thin walled and they contain one-way valves that prevent fluid from moving backward. They are like capillaries in that they have many holes between the endothelial cells, which make up their intimal layer. This allows the passage of fluid and small proteins from the interstitial space into the lymph vessels; they collect the fluid that accumulates in the interstitial space (having been filtered out, but not reabsorbed, from capillaries). This fluid is eventually returned by the lymphatics to the venous circulation via the right and left subclavian veins in the upper chest.

The Genesis of Edema: The Starling Forces

Under certain conditions, despite the presence of lymphatic vessels, more fluid leaks out of capillaries than can be either reabsorbed or collected by lymph vessels and returned to the circulation. The retention of fluid in the interstitial space is called "**edema**" (see *Figure* 8-5).

The physical forces that govern the movement of fluid (and proteins) into and out of capillaries are referred to as the "**Starling forces**," named after Ernest Starling, the man who first described them. There are two filtration forces and two reabsorption forces. Filtration forces promote movement of fluid out of capillaries and into the interstitial space that surrounds them. One of the two filtration forces is the fluid pressure within the capillary (called the **capillary hydrostatic pressure [CHP]**).

The second filtration force is a little less intuitive. When studying chemistry, you learned about osmotic pressure, the ability of particles on one side of a semipermeable membrane to create a force that draws fluid across it. Capillaries are surrounded by the interstitial space, which contain "particles" (large proteins) that are too big to cross the capillary membrane. The concentration of these particles leads to a force that enhances movement of water out of the capillary. This force is called the "**interstitial oncotic pressure**"; it constitutes the second, and much smaller, filtration pressure.

Reabsorptive forces draw fluid from the interstitial space back into the capillaries. As with the filtration, hydrostatic and oncotic forces come into play; in this case, however, the direction of the force is in the opposite direction, that is, facilitating movement of fluid from the interstitial space into the capillary. The oncotic pressure within the capillary is the consequence of the presence of large proteins *within the capillaries* (these proteins, such as albumin, are too large to cross the wall of the capillary); this is called the "**capillary oncotic pressure (COP).**" The hydrostatic force within the interstitial space is due to the pressure created by the buildup of fluid within this space; this is called "**interstitial hydrostatic pressure**" and it promotes fluid reentering the capillaries.

Now we will put all of these forces together to explain how they interact to prevent edema formation <u>in the healthy person.</u> Let's start with what happens along the length of a normal capillary. We will make it simpler by ignoring the interstitial oncotic and hydrostatic pressures (under normal conditions, there are relatively few proteins in the interstitial space, and the space has a very high compliance; hence, it is characterized by low hydrostatic and oncotic pressure) (*Figure* 8-5). Thus, we are left with one filtration force (CHP) and one reabsorptive force (COP).

Capillaries have both an arterial end and a venous end. At the arterial end, the CHP is around 35 mm Hg and the COP is slightly lower, say 28 mm Hg. Since the filtration force is greater than the reabsorptive force, there is net movement of fluid out of the capillary (filtration) and into the interstitial space. As you move along the normal capillary toward the venous end, the ratio of filtration to reabsorptive forces reverses. This is largely due to the fact that CHP falls along the length of the capillary from arterial to venous end. There is a natural loss of energy (in the form of pressure) as the flowing blood overcomes friction imposed by the surrounding walls. In addition, as the fluid leaves the capillary, the concentration of proteins remaining in the capillary increases; this has the effect of increasing COP. At the point along the capillary where the reabsorptive forces exceed the filtration forces, fluid reenters the capillary from the interstitial space (reabsorption). Under normal conditions, the fluid that is filtered is somewhat (but not perfectly) matched to the fluid that is reabsorbed. Any excess fluid that is left behind in the

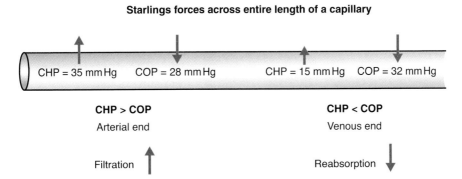

Starlings forces across entire length of a capillary

CHP = 35 mm Hg   COP = 28 mm Hg   CHP = 15 mm Hg   COP = 32 mm Hg

CHP > COP   **CHP < COP**
Arterial end   Venous end

Filtration   Reabsorption

FIGURE 8-5 Starling forces in a normal capillary. This figure illustrates the two forces, filtration and reabsorption, that determine the movement of fluid across the walls of a capillary as blood flows from arteriole to venule. Under normal conditions, the principal force of filtration is capillary hydrostatic pressure (CHP). The principal force of reabsorption is capillary oncotic pressure (COP). When CHP is more than COP (as at the arteriole end), net filtration occurs. When CHP is less than COP (as at the venule end), net reabsorption occurs.

interstitial space is easily mopped up by the lymph vessels and returned to the venous circulation.

When these forces are altered, edema, that is, excessive fluid in the interstitial space, may result. Normal reabsorption of fluid back into the capillary relies on a fall in CHP from the arterial to venous end of the capillary, such that it is less than the reabsorptive COP at the venous end of the capillary. If venous CHP remains high for any reason, it can exceed the COP along the entire length of the capillary; fluid is filtered into the interstitial space and not reabsorbed. If the volume of filtered fluid overwhelms the ability of the lymph system to remove it from the interstitial space, then fluid accumulates in the interstitial space and is called edema. When edema in the subcutaneous tissue is significant, you can press your finger against the skin and create an indentation or "pit" as you push the fluid away from the small region under your finger; when you pull your finger away from the skin, the indentation remains. We describe this physical exam finding as "pitting edema" (*Figure* 8-6).

The accumulation of edema fluid in other parts of the body may not be readily apparent by looking at a person but can cause symptoms such as shortness of breath (pulmonary edema) and conditions such as malabsorption (edema in the intestines).

Use Animated Figure 8-1 (Starling forces) to explore the forces governing filtration and reabsorption along the length of an idealized systemic capillary. Under normal conditions, filtration and reabsorption are reasonably well balanced, with lymphatic drainage taking care of any excess filtered fluid. Select "congestive heart failure" in the figure and observe the change in filtration accompanying the rise in CHP. Heart failure may lead to higher pressures in capillaries "upstream" of the failing ventricle; if the right ventricle is impaired, for example, the capillaries of the legs may experience higher hydrostatic pressures. In the figure, you can see that the pressure change favors filtration and, hence, edema if the extra filtration overwhelms the lymphatics' drainage capacity. Select "hypoproteinemia" (low protein in the blood) in the figure to see how a decrease in COP affects fluid movement. Here, too, edema may be the result, but due to a different alteration in Starling forces.

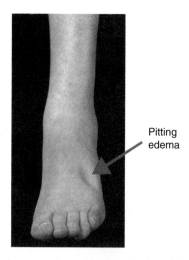

Pitting edema

FIGURE 8-6 Pitting edema. This image shows a patient with edema in the ankle and foot. A thumb pressed into the foot leaves a temporary depression, or pit, in the tissue as a result of the edema. This condition is called "pitting edema" and is due to increased venous hydrostatic pressures and/or decreased serum protein (and concomitant decreased oncotic pressure). Reprinted with permission from Bickley LS. *Bate's Guide to Physical Examination and History Taking.* 8th Ed. Philadelphia, PA: Lippincott Williams & Wilkins, 2003.

Vascular Resistance

EXCITATION–CONTRACTION COUPLING IN VASCULAR SMOOTH MUSCLE

Excitation–contraction (EC) coupling in vascular smooth muscle is not dissimilar to EC coupling in cardiac muscle (see *Figure* 3-3 and animated *Figure* 3-1 in Chapter 3). In both situations, a calcium–calmodulin complex phosphorylates the myosin light chain (MLC) heads by MLC kinase (MLCK), which allows cross-bridge formation between myosin and actin and leads to contraction. Contraction of the vascular smooth muscle (called vaso-constriction) reduces a vessel's radius and, according to Pouiselle's equation:

$$Flow = \Delta P \cdot r^4 / \eta \cdot L$$

where P is vessel pressure, r is vessel radius, η is blood viscosity and L is vessel length.

Thus, small decreases in radius result in large increases in resistance to blood flow. When the vasoconstriction is widespread in the body's vascular beds, it leads to an increase in systemic vascular resistance and elevation in blood pressure (BP = CO × SVR). Vaso-constrictive agents such as angiotensin II, vasopressin, and endothelin (released locally from vascular endothelial cells) act to initiate vascular smooth muscle contraction, reduce the radius of blood vessels, increase resistance, and thereby regulate blood pressure.

Other agonists, such as NO, act as powerful vasodilators. NO results in the generation of cGMP, which phosphorylates MLCK, rendering it incapable of phosphorylating MLC; this prevents actin–myosin cross-bridge formation in the muscle surrounding arterioles and, thereby, leads to vasodilation. NO-induced vasodilation is a local (as opposed to systemic) response; therefore, it does not contribute to a fall in systemic vascular resistance. The half-life of NO in the circulation is very short. Consequently, its actions are restricted to the vessels in the immediate region where it is released.

FACTORS THAT INFLUENCE VASCULAR DIAMETER

Systemic vascular resistance is the result of the ongoing balance between vasoconstriction and vasodilation (*Figure* 8-7). A number of factors influence this balance. They can be categorized into distant factors and local factors. Distant factors, either chemicals or conditions, produce constriction or dilation, arise externally to the vessels, and can act at a distance from where the chemical or condition arises. Local factors are chemicals or conditions inherent to the vascular smooth muscle that act close to where the chemical or condition originates. Distant factors include nerves (sympathetic and parasympathetic nerves) and hormones (angiotensin and vasopressin). Local factors include substances produced within the endothelial cells that line blood vessels (e.g., endothelin and NO), byproducts of tissue metabolism (e.g., adenosine, low oxygen, potassium), and a property of vascular smooth muscle called the "myogenic reflex." In each case, the local factor acts on vessels in the immediate region in which they are initiated.

Distant Control

As we just noted, distant control of vascular tone refers to circumstances in which substances or conditions that originate distant from the vessel act on the vascular smooth

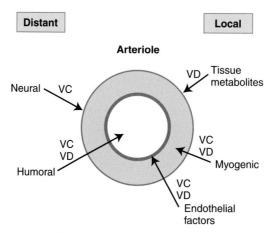

FIGURE 8-7 Local and distant vasoactive factors. This figure depicts the balance between factors that lead to vasoconstriction (VC) versus those that vasodilate (VD) blood vessels. These factors can be categorized as distant or local based on the proximity between the site at which the factor is initiated and the blood vessels upon which the factor exerts its effect.

muscle to alter its diameter. This category can be divided into two subcategories: neural or humoral.

Neural. Sympathetic nerves actively control vascular diameter and vascular resistance, and therefore, have a role to play in controlling blood pressure. Sympathetic nerves release the adrenergic neurotransmitter norepinephrine (also known as noradrenaline), which acts predominantly on α_1 postjunctional receptors on vascular smooth muscle cells (it also stimulates β_1-receptors in the heart, which leads to an increase in contractility of the myocytes). These receptors are mainly coupled to a Gq/11 protein that stimulates the enzyme phospholipase C, inositol trisphosphate (IP3), and diacylglycerol. IP3 binds to specific receptors on the sarcoplasmic reticulum and releases calcium. It's the rise in Ca^{2+} that activates MLCK and contraction. You may remember, however, that activation of the sympathetic limb of the autonomic nervous system also releases epinephrine (also known as adrenaline) from the adrenal gland into the blood stream. Epinephrine travels to the blood vessels and acts predominantly on β_2-receptors on vascular smooth muscle cells. β_2-receptor activation generates cAMP-dependent protein kinase (or PKA), which phosphorylates MLCK. This inactivates MLCK and thus interrupts contraction, thereby leading to vasodilation. As you can see, the α_1- and β_2-receptors create a balance between vasoconstriction and vasodilatation.

EDITOR'S INTEGRATION
This concept of regulating physiological function by the action of two opposing neurological stimuli is not unique to blood vessels. The diameter of the medium-size airways of the lung is controlled by the tone of the muscles surrounding the airways (much as the diameter of blood vessels is determined by the muscular tone of the arteries). The state of contraction of these muscles is determined by the balance of SNS activity, which causes bronchodilation, and parasympathetic activity, which leads to constriction of the airways.

A second alpha-receptor, alpha 2, found on the vascular smooth muscle, contributes further to this balance. Alpha 2 receptors are located on vascular smooth muscle cells, and when stimulated by NE cause vasoconstriction. In addition, however, there are alpha 2 receptors on the sympathetic nerve terminals themselves (called prejunctional receptors). Stimulation of the prejunctional receptors inhibits further norepinephrine release, thereby acting as a braking mechanism on vasoconstriction.

Endothelin-Induced Contraction

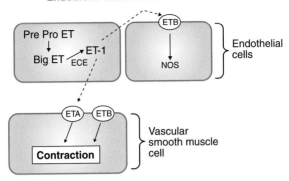

FIGURE 8-10 Endothelin mechanism of action. Endothelin 1 (ET-1) is synthesized from a precursor, big endothelin (ET), in the presence of endothelin-converting enzyme (ECE). ET-1 acts on ETA receptors on vascular smooth muscle cells to produce vasoconstriction. ET-1 also activates ETB receptors, which stimulate the release of nitric oxide synthase (NOS) leading to production of NO. Thus, the endothelial cell has an important role in balancing vasoconstriction and vasodilation. (Adapted from Smooth Muscle 06 handout. www.med-ed.virginia.edu)

arterial blood is directed away from poorly ventilated parts of the lungs to regions receiving ample oxygen, thereby maximizing oxygen uptake.

Special Circulations

CORONARY CIRCULATION

Coronary blood flow, like cerebral blood flow, is subject to autoregulation. Over the physiological range of pressures (approximately 60 to 160 mm Hg), despite increases in perfusion pressure, coronary blood flow is maintained constant. The mechanisms that contribute to this phenomenon include endothelium-mediated (**shear stress** activated) release of NO, the myogenic response, and thirdly, metabolically mediated release of NO. If cardiac muscle contractility and/or cardiac metabolism increase, however, metabolic vasodilators (adenosine, low pH, low oxygen) appear, which also lead to release of NO. This promotes an increase in coronary blood flow and contributes to a shift up in the autoregulatory plateau.

What makes coronary blood flow unique is that it is functionally linked to the cardiac cycle. During the powerful left ventricular systolic contraction, coronary arterial inflow is decreased and coronary venous outflow is increased. Effectively, therefore, left coronary perfusion occurs only during diastolic relaxation. This "systolic flow deficit" has implications for states in which diastolic filling time is substantially reduced; for example, a patient with severe narrowing of the aortic valve (aortic stenosis) and a thick, hypertrophied left ventricle may develop angina when HR is elevated.

It is also important to differentiate between the perfusion of the **epicardial** tissue (closest to the outer surface) and **endocardial** tissue (closest to the lumen). Since the coronary vessels penetrate into the cardiac muscle from their position on the surface of the heart, the *subendocardial* cells are the farthest distance away and experience the greatest drop in perfusion pressure as blood flows from the epicardial vessels. This makes them more susceptible to ischemia. Blood flow to the subendocardial cells is also dependent upon the intraventricular pressure during diastole; the perfusion pressure (ΔP) to this region of the heart is the BP in the blood vessel minus the intraventricular pressure. Patients with decreased compliance of the left ventricle, which is typically associated with high intraventricular pressures, are at particular risk of subendocardial ischemia.

? **THOUGHT QUESTION 8-5:** Given what you now know about left coronary artery perfusion during systole, what would you predict for right coronary perfusion during systole and diastole? If right ventricle pressures rise (due to pulmonary hypertension, for example), what do you think would happen to right coronary artery (RCA) perfusion?

? **THOUGHT QUESTION 8-6:** A person with a significantly narrowed lumen of a major coronary artery and cardiac hypertrophy consumes several high caffeine beverages that result in repeated episodes of angina. What would you predict would be the mechanism behind the generation of angina in this person?

CEREBRAL CIRCULATION

Like the coronary bed, the cerebral circulation is influenced by the interactions of humoral, neural, and metabolic factors, and is autoregulated. There are, however, several unique characteristics that govern cerebrovascular regulation. First, the cerebral vascular bed is enclosed in the skull, thus, changes in intracranial pressure influence cerebral perfusion pressure. Second, active regions in the brain alter vascular caliber to facilitate regional increases in blood flow. Let's look at each of the regulators of the cerebral vasculature in turn.

As we have seen in our discussions of blood flow to muscles, a key determinant of cerebral blood flow regulation is the generation of metabolic vasodilatory byproducts from active cerebral tissue. These include a range of substances and conditions such as potassium, adenosine, low O_2, high CO_2, NO, and lactate. The more active the brain tissue, the more vasodilatory substances are generated; this results in more blood flow to that area. Studies investigating metabolic control of cerebral blood flow have demonstrated distinct areas of the brain that showed increased blood flow in the context of particular intellectual tasks (reasoning, problem solving) and in response to behavioral tasks (visual and auditory).

The cerebral circulation can also be affected by some of the systemic regulators of vascular tone. Several humoral vasoactive substances (e.g., vasopressin and angiotensin) access the cerebral circulation via cerebral areas devoid of the **blood–brain barrier** (e.g., choroid plexus) and exert vasoactive effects on the cerebral circulation.

Although the cerebral vasculature is richly innervated with autonomic nerve fibers, sympathetic nerve stimulation has little net effect on cerebral blood flow. This observation is due, in part, to the fact that sympathetic-induced constriction in large cerebral arteries is offset by autoregulatory dilation in small arterioles; thus, there is no net change in blood flow. Sympathetic stimulation, however, may have an important role in protecting the brain from hypertension; in this case, sympathetic-induced vasoconstriction of cerebral vessels may attenuate increases in cerebral blood flow due to hypertension. Parasympathetic innervation of cerebral vasculature also exists, but its physiological role in regulating cerebral blood flow is unclear.

PULMONARY CIRCULATION

The pulmonary vascular bed is a low resistance system in which the normal arteriovenous pressure difference is approximately 10 mm Hg (compared with ~90 mm Hg in the systemic vascular bed). This low resistance is accounted for, in part, by the vasodilatory action of NO, which promotes low basal vascular tone and leads to receptor-mediated (acetylcholine, bradykinin, substance P, serotonin, and ATP) vasodilation. In contrast to the systemic vasculature, autonomic (sympathetic and parasympathetic) stimulation has a minimal effect on the regulation of the pulmonary vasculature, although the SNS may have a role in maintenance of normal pulmonary vascular tone. Another big difference from systemic vessels is that low tissue oxygen (e.g., PO_2 below 50 mm Hg), in this case represented by alveolar oxygen levels, produces brisk, sustained pulmonary vasoconstriction. This makes sense physiologically since vasoconstriction in the context of low oxygen leads to redirection of blood away from underventilated areas of the lung and (hopefully) toward better-ventilated areas where fresh oxygen can be picked up and carbon dioxide can be offloaded. The mechanism behind the hypoxic stimulation of vasoconstriction may be an inhibition of K^+ current in vascular smooth muscle resulting in membrane depolarization, generation of action potentials, and vasoconstriction; ET-1 may also play a role.

You should remember from anatomy that the tissue of the lung receives oxygen to sustain its metabolic activity via the bronchial arteries, which arise from the aorta, from oxygen in the airways and alveoli, and from the pulmonary arteries. Thus, if blood in the pulmonary arteries is redirected away from regions with low oxygen levels, this usually does not cause harm to the lung tissue. The primary purpose of the pulmonary arteries is to pick up oxygen from the alveoli for delivery to the rest of the body.

Angiogenesis

First, let's distinguish between two important terms that refer to the genesis of new blood vessels. In the embryo, a primitive vascular network is established by the de novo production of endothelial cells, which are then associated with smooth muscle cells, pericytes, and macrophages. This process is called "**vasculogenesis**" (development of new blood vessels from precursor cells). Subsequently, these primitive vessels undergo budding and branching and this process is referred to as "**angiogenesis**" (development of new blood vessels from preexisting vessels). Under a variety of physiological situations, this combined process of vasculogenesis and angiogenesis continues throughout your adult life.

We will review the basic steps that drive the process of angiogenesis. Initially, the walls of the endothelial cell basement membrane (in the existing vessels) must be broken down. This is followed by activation and proliferation of quiescent endothelial cells, which then migrate into the extracellular matrix to form a new endothelial tube. Pericytes, macrophages, and smooth muscle cells are subsequently attracted to the endothelial tube to complete the new vessel. Ultimately, the newly formed vessels must be "sealed" within a new extracellular matrix. This entire process represents a delicate balance between the synthesis and release of **proangiogenic** and **antiangiogenic** factors. Proangiogenic growth factors include primarily heparin-binding substances such as basic fibroblast growth factor (bFGF), vascular endothelial growth factor (VEGF), the insulin-like growth factor (IGF) system, and HIF-1α. Naturally occurring antiangiogenic factors include angiostatin and endostatin.

Inappropriate angiogenesis can contribute to various disease states; prominent among these conditions is the increase in vessels seen in rapidly growing cancers. Tumors under 2 cm in diameter can continue to sustain nourishment from existing microcirculation. With increasing tumor growth, however, the interior cells become increasingly hypoxic. This stimulates proangiogenic growth factors and facilitates the process of tumor angiogenesis (*Figure* 8-11). There has been much research into targeting tumor angiogenesis as a way to combat tumor development. To slow vascular growth, you can either inhibit naturally occurring proangiogenic factors (e.g., VEGF, IGF, etc.) or you can treat with exogenous antiangiogenic substances (e.g., angiostatin and endostatin among others).

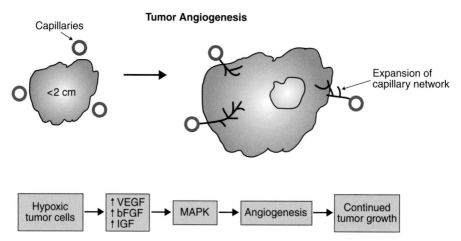

Tumor Angiogenesis

FIGURE 8-11 Tumor angiogenesis. This figure illustrates that tumors under 2 cm in diameter can acquire sufficient blood supply from surrounding capillaries. Tumors greater than 2 cm in diameter may develop hypoxic cores that stimulate the release of proangiogenic factors (VEGF, bFGF, and IGF) and, hence, encourage the process of tumor-induced angiogenesis. Adapted from Gupta MK, Qin RY. Mechanism and its regulation of tumor-induced angiogenesis. *World J Gastroenterol* 2003; 9(6): 1144–1155.

? **THOUGHT QUESTION 8-7:** **What does formation of the placenta in a pregnant woman have in common with exercise training? Why would you expect this?**

PUTTING IT TOGETHER

While waiting to board a bus you notice the woman standing beside you; she looks to be in her sixties and seems very anxious. All of a sudden, she drops her briefcase, clutches her chest, and sinks to her knees. Her name is Katherine and when you reach her she is sweating and looks terrified. She is having trouble breathing and she says she feels like there is sharp, burning sensation in her chest. Once in the ambulance and lying quietly while breathing supplemental oxygen, Katherine's chest pain resolves. The feeling of burning in her chest has happened several times previously in stressful situations at work. The pain is relieved when she removes herself from the situation and rests for 10 minutes. What physiological factors could account for her chest pain?

What Katherine is experiencing is called "angina pectoris," which is the term for chest pain associated with myocardial ischemia and relieved by rest or nitroglycerin. Under normal conditions of rest and minimal exertion, the blood supplied by Katherine's coronary arteries is adequate to meet her metabolic demands (supply = demand). Within the context of mentally or emotionally stressful situations, however, the demand placed on her heart muscle is increased beyond what is being supplied by her coronary arteries and, thus, she experiences myocardial ischemia (demand > supply). The question before you is: What is causing her diminished coronary blood supply? It could be narrowing of her coronary artery(ies) as a result of deposition of atherosclerotic plaques. This could be determined by employing techniques that image her coronary arteries (angiography). It would be useful to determine her cholesterol/triglyceride profile to see whether she is above the normal levels. High blood cholesterol increases her risk factor for coronary artery disease.

Alternatively, the use of drugs, such as cocaine, can stimulate vasospasm with severe narrowing of the coronary vessels, which leads to high vascular resistance and reduced flow. In some patients, coronary spasm can occur spontaneously. An increase in myocardial oxygen demand, as occurs during stress (increased sympathetic stimulation), tachycardia, and exercise,

poorly responsive to two strong hormonal vasoconstrictors, angiotensin II and norepinephrine. Additionally, the endothelial cells lining the vasculature may contribute to the vasodilatory state by increasing release of two powerful vasodilators, prostacyclin and nitric oxide (see Chapter 8, "Blood Vessels"). To date, no link between estrogen and progesterone (two important hormones of pregnancy) and the vasodilatory state can be conclusively made. Progesterone is a smooth muscle relaxant and may contribute to vasodilatation through this mechanism.

EDITOR'S INTEGRATION
Progesterone's action on smooth muscle is felt to contribute to the symptom of heartburn that accompanies gastroesophageal reflux, a common complication of pregnancy. A muscle called the lower esophageal sphincter regulates the movement of food and liquid at the junction between the esophagus and the stomach. When the muscle relaxes, acid from the stomach can reflux into the esophagus, which causes a substernal burning sensation.

? **THOUGHT QUESTION 10-3:** How might you explain the observation that in the face of increased plasma volume in pregnant women, plasma renin concentration is slightly elevated, whereas plasma atrial natriuretic peptide is slightly reduced?

Cardiovascular Events Associated with Labor and Delivery

As you might expect, there are some particularly dramatic cardiovascular changes associated with labor and delivery. Systolic blood pressure varies in association with uterine contractions during labor, in part related to maternal body position, intensity or stage of labor, and the anxiety levels experienced by the laboring woman. Women in the supine position experience exaggerated changes in arterial pressure and cardiac output primarily as a result of compression of the inferior vena cava by the contracting uterus. By adjusting the mother's position from the supine to the left lateral decubitus position (lying on her left side), one can minimize this effect. Uterine contractions (and the associated anxiety and pain) increase sympathetic nervous system activity, which results in increased maternal cardiac output and blood pressure. In addition, there is an internal transfusion of blood from the uterine sinusoids to the material circulation that occurs during active labor; consequently, there is an increase in cardiac preload and blood pressure with each contraction (see Chapter 7).

During the pushing stage of labor, there may be transient hypotensive periods similar to what is seen during Valsalva maneuver; when one squeezes the chest with the glottis closed, intrathoracic pressure rises, venous return falls and, thus, blood pressure falls after a short period of time. In pregnant women with a normal autonomic nervous system, this triggers a baroreflex and causes maternal tachycardia. Hypotension during labor may be influenced by body position as described previously.

Immediately following delivery, cardiac output is increased by an astounding 80% compared to prelabor levels; this is observed despite the sudden drop in anxiety, pain, and the cessation of muscular efforts associated with contractions and pushing. The rise in cardiac output postpartum is due largely to the autotransfusion of blood from the utero/placental unit to the maternal circulation (as described above).

Cardiac Examination During Pregnancy

The commonly seen cardiovascular adaptations to pregnancy are reflected in the cardiac examination of the pregnant woman. Of course, the magnitude of the observed changes varies from the beginning to the end of pregnancy. Examination of the chest may reveal a shift in the **apical impulse** (felt when the apex of the heart thrusts against the chest wall during systolic contraction), reflecting a shift in the heart's position in the thorax as the enlarging uterus pushes against the diaphragm and moves the heart into a more horizontal (transverse) position. Auscultation of the heart may reveal the appearance of a louder first heart sound (AV valves closing), which is likely due to the elevated heart rate (which results in more rapid valve leaflet closure during diastole; see Chapter 4) and higher cardiac output. A third heart sound is a common finding in pregnant women and is most likely due to increased intravascular volume. The high cardiac output and low viscosity state of pregnancy may result in a murmur heard in conjunction with systolic contraction.

> ### EDITOR'S INTEGRATION
> *Pregnancy is also associated with changes in the respiratory examination. The increased abdominal girth leads to elevation of the diaphragm, which can be assessed by percussing the chest (tapping on the chest with your fingers). Despite the elevated diaphragm, the size of each breath, called the tidal volume, is preserved. The total amount of air breathed each minute (minute ventilation) is increased; progesterone stimulates breathing and increases ventilation leading to a respiratory alkalosis (low $PaCO_2$ and high pH).*

Fetal/Neonatal Transition

In addition to the adaptations the cardiovascular system must make in the mother to support the metabolic needs of the pregnancy, the system must also accommodate the needs of the fetus, which is functionally bound to the maternal circulatory system. The maternal placenta supplies the fetus with freshly oxygenated blood that returns, via the umbilical vein, to the fetal heart and passes through a unidirectional flap in the interatrial septum, called the foramen ovale (forming a right to left shunt). After passing through the foramen ovale, the oxygenated blood flows into the left atrium. The existence of the foramen allows blood to go directly from right to left atrium, thus, bypassing the, as yet, nonfunctional (fluid filled) fetal lungs (*Figure* 10-6). The right to left shunt through the foramen ovale is possible since the pressure in the fetal right atrium is higher than the left atrium. This pressure differential in the fetal heart is the result of normal venous return to the right atrium from the body combining with the flow from the umbilical vein, which greatly exceeds the pressure generated by small volume of blood coming back to the left atrium from the fetal lungs. The blood in the left atrium—a combination now of umbilical vein, vena caval, and pulmonary venous blood—passes into the left ventricle and out through the aorta to the fetal systemic circulation.

Some deoxygenated blood does not go through the foramen ovale; it returns from the head and neck via the superior vena cava and passes into the right ventricle from where it is pumped into the pulmonary arteries. Fetal pulmonary vascular resistance is very high (fetal pulmonary arterioles are mostly closed; there is no oxygen in the lung, and hypoxic pulmonary vasoconstriction results), thus blood in the main pulmonary artery is diverted through a second fetal shunt; this one is between the pulmonary artery and the aorta and is called the "ductus arteriosus." As a result of this shunt, some deoxygenated blood from the ductus mixes in the aorta with the freshly oxygenated blood that passed through the foramen ovale. Despite this mixing of oxygenated and deoxygenated blood, the oxygen saturation of the mixed blood is still sufficiently high to supply the needs of the fetus.

Animated Figure 10-1 shows you the path of blood through the fetal circulation. Notice how the two shunts described above—the foramen ovale and the ductus arteriosus—allow blood to bypass the fetal lungs.

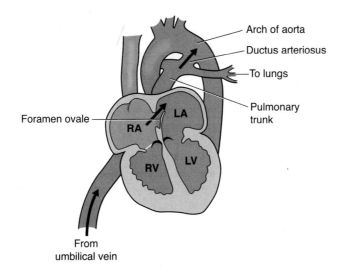

Arch of aorta

Ductus arteriosus

To lungs

Pulmonary trunk

Foramen ovale

LA

RA

RV

LV

From umbilical vein

FIGURE 10-6 Fetal circulation. Two principal cardiac shunts exist in order to facilitate the fetal access to oxygenated blood in the face of not-yet-functional lungs. Oxygenated blood from the placenta flows into the right atrium (RA) via the umbilical vein and the inferior vena cava (IVC) and passes directly through to the left atrium (LA) via the first shunt, called the foramen ovale. The second shunt allows mixed (oxygenated/deoxygenated) blood to flow from the pulmonary artery (PA) directly into the aorta through the ductus arteriosus.

At birth there is an abrupt change in the fetal cardiac circulation. The baby takes its first breath, the lungs fill with air, alveolar hypoxia is relieved, and the pulmonary arterioles open and fill with blood, thus dropping the pulmonary vascular resistance. At the same time, the umbilical arteries constrict and the umbilical cord is severed; the source of oxygenated blood now switches from the placenta to the baby's lungs. The fall in pulmonary vascular resistance lowers the right atrial pressure, whereas the increased venous return from the lungs to the left atrium raises the left atrial pressure; this combination of events reverses the interatrial pressure gradient seen in the fetus and closes the foramen ovale. Blood in the right atrium now flows into the right ventricle, through the pulmonary circulation and back to the left atrium. At birth, a combination of higher concentrations of oxygen in the blood and withdrawal of placental vasodilating prostaglandins results in vasoconstriction of the ductus arteriosus, thereby closing the communication between the main pulmonary artery and the aorta. The neonate now has two completely separate arterial and venous circulations flowing in series through the heart, a circulation that will sustain the body for the rest of its life.

 The second part of Animated Figure 10-1, seen when you initiate the birth transition, illustrates the changes that allow the remarkable reconfiguration of the fetal circulation at birth. As discussed, the two shunts (foramen ovale and ductus arteriosus) close off because of the oxygenation of the lungs, and the changes in pulmonary vascular resistance and interatrial pressure difference. Notice the difference in the circulation prebirth and postbirth; the placental source of oxygenated blood is removed and the lungs are included in the circuit.

THOUGHT QUESTION 10-4: Newborn babies can exhibit transient cyanosis (blue cast to skin and mucous membranes) when crying or straining. From what you know about fetal neonatal transition, what could explain these transient periods of cyanosis?

PUTTING IT TOGETHER

Carlos and Teresa are expecting their first child. Teresa, who has gained a healthy 10.8 kg (approximately 25% of her prepregnancy weight), is half way through her third trimester (~32 weeks) and beginning to find it difficult to achieve a comfortable position in which to relax. One evening, while lying on her couch and watching a movie, she shifts her position from lying on her left side to lying on her back. Within several minutes, she notices her pulse is racing and she feels anxious and lightheaded. She calls out to Carlos. Assuming she is not watching a scary movie, what can account for the change in Teresa's cardiovascular findings?

What she is experiencing is symptomatic positional hypotension, also known as supine hypotensive syndrome. As the uterus grows in size to accommodate the growing fetus, it may press down on the maternal inferior vena cava (IVC) in the supine position. Compression of the IVC limits venous return, such that there is a transient fall in blood pressure, which activates the arterial baroreceptors. Less stretch on the baroreceptors results in disinhibition of the sympathetic nerves, with release of norepinephrine as the nerves are activated, which results in a profound tachycardia, increased inotropy, and vasoconstriction (increased SVR). During the period prior to restoration of normal blood pressure, there is a subjective feeling of anxiety and lightheadedness, which may be accompanied by restlessness, nausea, and other symptoms of hypotension. These symptoms can be relieved by having the woman roll on to her left side (called the left lateral decubitus position). This displaces the uterus to the left and off the IVC.

Summary Points

- To meet the needs of the developing fetus, maternal blood volume increases and blood viscosity decreases, that is, plasma volume increases more than red blood cell mass.
- The changes in maternal blood characteristics facilitate fetal perfusion and exchange of nutrients and wastes, while minimizing the increase in maternal cardiac work.
- Because the increase in maternal red blood cell mass is less pronounced than the increase in plasma volume, the hematocrit is lower. The reduced hematocrit is characterized as "physiological anemia." Oxygen delivery, the product of the oxygen content of the blood and the cardiac output, is maintained.
- Maternal cardiac output is elevated as a result of increases in both stroke volume and heart rate.
- The increase in cardiac output reflects an increase in maternal preload and a decrease in SVR; the latter results from peripheral vasodilatation and increased vascular capacity.
- Because of the influence of hormones during pregnancy, there is an increase in the capacitance (dilation) of the large veins of the legs, and a state of hypercoagulability. Together these create a milieu that predisposes the mother to the development of deep vein thrombosis and pulmonary embolism.
- Maternal SVR falls during pregnancy. Consequently, despite the high cardiac output, blood pressure is either unchanged or slightly lowered in a normal pregnancy (the change in BP is the result of an ↑CO and decrease in ↓SVR; if the two are balanced, systemic BP may not be altered).
- Maternal vasodilation may be the result of reduced responsiveness of the mother's blood vessels to two strong hormonal vasoconstrictors, angiotensin II and norepinephrine. In addition, the endothelial hormones, nitric oxide and prostacyclin, may play a role in the fall in SVR.
- The creation of the utero/placental unit is the consequence of a combination of vasculogenesis and angiogenesis.

tachycardia, lightheadedness, and anxiety. Her anemia is likely physiological due to an unbalanced increase in plasma volume versus red blood cell mass. SVR decreases rather than increases with pregnancy. Also, her symptoms are related to specific posture that makes hypovolemia (options A and B) unlikely. The maternal blood volume increases in pregnancy, not decreases, thus option D is incorrect.

10-4. **C.** During birth, the decrease in pulmonary resistance with the first breath combines with increased pulmonary venous return to the left atrium to reverse the pressure differential that had favored flow from right to left atrium in the fetus; left atrial pressure now exceeds right atrial pressure, and if the atrial septal defect (ASD) persists after birth, it leads to a **left-to-right** shunt. In this case, oxygenated blood returning from the lungs to the left atrium travels to the right atrium, right ventricle, and back to the lungs. To see cyanosis, you would need to have a right-to-left shunt of deoxygenated blood returning from the body, flowing across the interatrial septum and, finally, entering the systemic circulation without passing through the lungs. Option B is not correct, as the closure (at birth) of the ductus arteriosus does not allow mixing of oxygenated and deoxygenated blood between the aorta and the pulmonary artery. Option D is not correct as fetal hemoglobin binds oxygen more tightly than does neonatal (and adult) hemoglobin. This does not contribute to cyanosis, which reflects only the quantity of deoxygenated hemoglobin; deoxygenated hemoglobin does not change.

Glossary of Terms

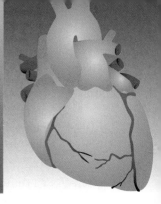

Action potential: In the context of the heart, this refers to the change in membrane potential that occurs in the cardiac muscle cell as the result of electrical excitation.

Adrenergic receptors: Receptors for epinephrine (adrenaline) or norepinephrine (noradrenaline) that are activated during excitation of the sympathetic nervous system.

Afferent: From the Latin "to bring towards," as in nerves bringing information from peripheral receptors toward the brain (where the information is processed).

Afterload: The tension in the ventricular wall (wall stress) necessary to generate the pressure required to open the aortic valve and eject the stroke volume.

Alveolar hypoxia: Low oxygen levels in the alveoli (air sacs) of the lung.

Anaerobic metabolism: Generation of energy in the absence of oxygen.

Angiogenesis: The process by which existing blood vessels undergo budding and branching, thereby extending the vascular tree.

Apical impulse: This is a pressure pulse palpated (felt by touching) at the apex (lowest superficial aspect) of the heart; this typically reflects contraction of the left ventricle.

Arterioles: Very small branches of the arterial tree that are smaller than arteries, but larger than capillaries.

Atria: Relatively thin walled, upper chambers of the heart that empty into the ventricles. The singular is atrium.

Atrial muscle cells: Cardiac muscle cells that make up the walls of the right and the left atrium.

Atrioventricular node: A cluster of pacemaker cells located at the bottom of the right atrium near the opening of the tricuspid valve. Under normal conditions, the electrical signal from the atrium to the ventricles must pass through the atrioventricular node.

Atrioventricular valves: A classification of heart valves that includes the tricuspid valve (between the right atrium and the right ventricle) and the mitral valve (between the left atrium and the left ventricle).

Autoregulation: The capacity of an organ to maintain a constant blood flow in the face of changes in blood pressure over a range of pressures (e.g., between 60 and 160 mm Hg). Flow is maintained via alterations in the resistance of the blood vessels supplying the organ.

Baroreceptors: Specialized stretch-sensitive nerve endings located in the walls of the aorta (called aortic arch baroreceptors) and at the bifurcation of the carotid arteries (called the carotid sinus baroreceptors). Alteration of the activity of the baroreceptors stimulates physiological responses to changes in blood pressure.

Bradycardia: Heart rate slower than 60 beats/min in adults.

Bulk flow: Movement of a liquid (e.g., plasma) across a membrane (e.g., capillary endothelium) in response to a difference in hydrostatic pressure, independent of solute concentration.

Calcium-induced calcium release: A mechanism in cardiac muscle cells whereby a small amount of calcium that enters the cell during depolarization facilitates release of calcium from the sarcoplasmic reticulum in sufficient concentration to allow cross-bridge cycling and contraction.

Capillaries: The smallest vessels, distal to arterioles and proximal to venules. Site of exchange of oxygen and carbon dioxide between vessels and the tissues they supply.

Cardiac controller: The elements of the cardiovascular system responsible for initiating the electrical activity necessary for cardiac contraction as well as for responding to changes in physiological parameters such as blood pressure.

Cardiac output: Volume of blood pumped from the ventricles each minute.

Cardiac myocyte: The cardiac muscle cell; contains myofibrils (actin and myosin), mitochondria, a sarcoplasmic reticulum, a system of transverse tubules (T tubules), and is bound by a cell membrane (sarcolemma).

Cardiac skeleton: A band of fibrous tissue, which forms rings around the atrioventricular, pulmonary, and aortic orifices (essentially the floor of the atria), that acts as an electrical insulator between the atria and the ventricles.

Central venous pressure: The blood pressure measured in the inferior or superior vena cava. Under normal conditions, the central venous pressure is an approximation of right atrial pressure.

Channelopathies: Refers to diseases that relate specifically to dysfunction of one or more ion channels; these conditions alter the action potential of the cardiac myocyte.

Chronotropy/chronotropic: From the Latin chrono (time) tropy (a change in response to a stimulus). Used in reference to a change in heart rate, either slower or faster.

Chordae tendineae: Cord-like small string-like structures located in the ventricles, attached on one end to the atrioventricular valve leaflets and on the other to small extensions of ventricular muscle called papillary muscles. These structures stabilize the valve leaflets during ventricular contraction.

Compliance: A measure of the distensibility (ratio of change in volume to change in pressure) of the heart chamber of the blood vessel. Units of compliance are mL/mm Hg.

Contractility: The strength of ventricular contraction at any given end-diastolic volume.

Coronary arteries: Arteries that originate from the aorta (just distal to the aortic annulus) and whose function is to supply the cardiac muscle with oxygen and nutrients.

Cross-bridge formation/cross-bridge cycling: Flexion of the myosin heads draws the actin fibrils along the myosin fibrils, thus shortening the cardiac muscle and generating tension. Cross-bridge formation requires the presence of calcium. Removal of calcium from the cytosol releases the cross-bridge and the cardiac muscle relaxes. This process of contraction and relaxation is called cross-bridge cycling.

Delayed rectifiers: Voltage-gated protein channels that are responsible for the movement of potassium across the cell membrane in all cardiac cells.

Depolarization: A rapid shift from negative to positive membrane potential that contributes to the generation of the action potential in cardiac cells.

Diastole: One of two phases of the cardiac cycle; diastole includes ventricular relaxation and filling.

Diastolic pressure: The arterial pressure measured between ventricular contractions.

Ectopic beats: A heartbeat whose origin is outside the normal conduction system.

Edema: An abnormal accumulation of fluid in the interstitial spaces between capillaries and surrounding tissue cells.

Efferent: From the Latin "to carry away," as in nerves carrying information from the brain to the periphery.

Ejection fraction: The fraction of left ventricular end-diastolic volume that is ejected as stroke volume. Calculated as $EF = (EDV - ESV)/EDV$.

Elastic recoil: Forces acting to return large arteries to their resting diameter in response to an increase in pressure; related to the presence of elastic tissue in the walls of the arteries. Helps maintain diastolic pressure in the arteries.

End-diastolic volume: The volume in the ventricle at the end of diastole; correlates with the "preload" of the ventricle.

Endothelin: A protein synthesized and released from endothelial cells; acts as a vasoconstrictor.

Endothelium (cardiac): The layer of cells that line the inside of the vessels (blood and lymphatic) and the heart chambers.

Endocardium/endocardial: From the Greek endo (inner) and cardium (heart), in reference to the innermost layer of endothelial cells that line the heart chambers.

End-systolic volume: The volume of the ventricle at the end of systole.

Epicardium/epicardial: From the Greek epi (outer) and cardium (heart), in reference to the outer layer of connective tissue covering the heart.

Exchanger: The elements of the cardiovascular system at which gases (oxygen and carbon dioxide) and nutrients are exchanged between the blood and the tissue; the capillaries.

Fixed splitting: A condition characterized by the absence of the normal change in the interval between the two components (A2, P2) of the second heart sound (S2) during the respiratory cycle.

Flow (e.g., blood): The volume of blood per unit time. As an example, the volume of blood that moves through the heart in one minute (called the cardiac output); measured in mL/min or L/min.

Gallop: The presence of third (or fourth) heart sound in addition to the normal first and second heart sounds (S1 and S2); results in a sound that resembles that of a galloping horse.

Gap junctions: Regions between adjacent cardiac cells that allow passage of action potentials from one cell to the next.

Hypertension: The medical term for chronic high blood pressure.

Hypertrophy: From the Latin "hyper" (excessive) "trophy" (growth). Enlargement of an organ or body part as a result of increased cell size or mass.

Hypotension: The medical term for low blood pressure. If associated with postural changes, for example, the transition from lying to standing, it is called "orthostatic hypotension."

Inotropy: From the Latin ino (fiber) tropy (a change in response to a stimulus). Used in reference to contractility or the ability to develop force at a given muscle fiber length.

Inward rectifier: A protein channel in the cardiac cell that moves potassium from outside to inside the cell. Action of the inward rectifier is important in establishing the configuration of the cardiac action potential, particularly the resting membrane potential.

Isovolumetric contraction/relaxation: The period during which both atrioventricular and semilunar valves are closed and pressure in the ventricle is either rising (isovolumetric contraction) or falling (isovolumetric relaxation). No blood is moving into or out of the ventricles during these periods.

Laminar blood flow: Smooth or streamlined blood flow in a heart chamber or through a blood vessel. Under laminar conditions, changes in flow are proportional to changes in driving pressure.

Lusitropy/lusitropic: Used in reference to relaxation of cardiac muscle.

Medulla: The most caudal subdivision of the brain stem. In conjunction with other cerebral structures, including the rostral ventrolateral medulla and the hypothalamus, it is referred to as the "cardiovascular control center."

Murmur: A sound heard during auscultation; the result of turbulent blood flow across a valve or through an opening between chambers.

Myocardial infarction: Necrosis of myocardial tissue due to interruption or impairment of oxygen (arterial narrowing or spasm).

Myocardial ischemia: Hypoxia of heart tissue due to transient interruption or impairment of oxygen delivery (arterial narrowing or spasm) relative to oxygen demand. If prolonged, it leads to myocardial infarction. Can be reversed with reperfusion or reduction in the metabolic needs of the myocardium.

Nernst equilibrium potential: The electrical potential that would exist if a cardiac cell membrane were selectively permeable to only one ion, and if the concentration gradient was equal and opposite to the electrical gradient.

Nitric oxide: A gas, the conversion product of L-arginine by nitric oxide synthase (NOS) in endothelial cells, that acts as a potent vasodilator.

P wave: The waveform on the ECG that represents atrial depolarization.

Pacemaker cells: Specialized cardiac muscle cells whose function is to initiate action potentials. These cells are characterized by an action potential with an upward slope to phase 4, which results in spontaneous depolarization.

Papillary muscle: Small finger-like extensions of ventricular muscle that are attached to chordae tendineae (see earlier). The action of the papillary muscle–chordae tendineae complex stabilizes the leaflets of the atrioventricular valves during systole.

Paradoxical splitting: When the two sounds of S2 (A2 and P2) are heard as distinct sounds during expiration and as one sound during inspiration (the opposite of physiological splitting).

Parasympathetic nervous system (PSNS): One of the limbs of the autonomic nervous system originating in the brain stem; stimulation of the PSNS slows the heart rate.

Pericardial sac: A fibroserous sac that encloses the heart and the beginning of the great vessels.

Pleural pressure: The pressure in the space between the visceral and parietal pleura. Under normal conditions, with quiet breathing, the pleural pressure is between -3 and -8 cm H_2O.

Preload: The length of the cardiac myocyte just before initiation of contraction. Preload is estimated from the end-diastolic volume of the ventricle, that is, prior to contraction.

Pulsus paradoxus: A transient decrease in blood pressure that is associated with inspiration during the respiratory cycle.

QRS wave: The waveform on the ECG that represents ventricular depolarization.

Refractory period: A defined period in the cardiac action potential during which the fast sodium channels are inactivated and unable to accept a new action potential.

Repolarization: A return from positive to negative membrane potential in the cardiac cell.

Sarcolemma: From the Greek sarco (flesh) and lemma (husk or shell). The cell membrane that encloses a myocardial cell.

Sarcomere: From the Greek sarco (flesh) and meros (part). The contractile unit of cardiac muscle; it contains action and myosin fibrils.

Sarcoplasmic reticulum: A net-like structure of vesicles (Latin "rete" for little net), cisternae, and tubules that surrounds each myofibril; structure in which calcium is stored between contractions.

Semilunar valves: A classification of heart valves that includes the pulmonic valve, located between the right ventricle and the pulmonary trunk, and the aortic valve, located between the left ventricle and the aorta.

Shear stress: The stress (force per unit area) resulting from the flow of blood applied tangentially to the luminal wall.

Sinoatrial node: A cluster of pacemaker cells located in the upper right corner of the right atrium at the junction with the superior vena cava. These cells are responsible for initiating the electrical activity responsible for cardiac contraction under normal conditions.

Skeletal muscle pump: The presence of skeletal muscles surrounding the veins in the legs; rhythmic contraction and relaxation of these muscles promotes blood flow returning to the heart.

Sodium channels: Voltage-sensitive protein channels that conduct sodium ions across the plasma membrane; they are responsible for the rapid upstroke (depolarization) in cardiac muscle cells.

Starling forces: The forces that, acting together, promote either fluid filtration from or reabsorption into capillaries. Hydrostatic forces favor filtration; oncotic forces favor reabsorption.

Stenotic valve: Refers to the narrowing of a heart valve orifice.

Sympathetic nervous system (SNS): One of the limbs of the autonomic nervous system, originating in the brain stem, that increases heart rate and the strength of myocardial contraction when activated.

Systemic vascular resistance (SVR): The total resistance of the vascular circuit; calculated from the equation: SVR = CO/(MAP − CVP). Provides an approximation of arterial constriction or dilation.

Systole: With respect to the cardiac cycle, systole represents ventricular contraction and ejection.

Systolic blood pressure: The arterial pressure measured at the peak of ventricular contraction.

T-tubules: Deep invaginations of the sarcolemma (plasma membrane) containing ion channels for calcium, sodium, and potassium; T-tubules are in close approximation to the sarcoplasmic reticulum in the cardiac muscle cell.

T wave: The waveform on the ECG that represents ventricular repolarization.

Tachycardia: Heart rate faster than 100 beats/min in adults.

Thoracic cavity: The space occupied by the lungs, the heart, and great vessels.

Turbulent blood flow: Flow in which the direction of movement of molecules of a fluid (in this case blood) is chaotic and not parallel to the main or overall direction of flow.

Unidirectional valve: A valve that allows fluid to pass in one direction but prevents the fluid from going in the opposite direction; in the heart, valve leaflet closure prevents backward flow.

Uterine sinusoids: Irregular vascular channels, filled with blood, that form in the uterine endometrium during pregnancy.

Vasoconstriction/venoconstriction: From the Latin "vas" for vessel and "constrigere" to tighten. The act of narrowing the blood vessel lumen as a consequence of the constriction of the smooth muscle in the media of the vessel wall.

Vasculogenesis: Establishment in the embryo of a primitive vascular network by the de novo production of endothelial cells, which are then associated with smooth muscle cells, pericytes, and macrophages.